# CONTENTS

# ACKNOWLEDGMENTS

**M**ANY THANKS to the countless people who lent me their time and expertise through often repeated and exhaustive interviews. For instance, Sandy Gooch, who makes it easier for people to find food to grow on at her chain of stores, shared with me many sources of expert knowledge. Much gratitude also goes to Steve Lederman, Dr. Lendon Smith, Wallace Sconier, Susan Harnett, Sarah L. Bingham, Virginia Young, Dr. Carol Port, Dr. Joyce Virtue, Dr. Paul Fleiss, Dr. Michael Jacobson, Dr. Judith Anderson, Karen McIntosh, Mary Queen, Betty Carl, and Anastasia Condas.

Special tribute goes to Dr. Bart Asner, who shepherded me through the care of our first two children, and Dr. Graydon Funke, whose words have counselled many parents. Recognition is also extended to Dr. Michael Sussman for his East Coast review. Other invaluable support has come from La Leche League, both in my interviews with co-founder Marian Thompson, and from the local Saddleback Valley and South Bay chapters.

I'd also like to thank Sean for giving his mom (Deborah Burns, my editor at Storey) a personal reason for believing in this book. Similar gratitude goes to Olivia, daughter of agent Deborah Schneider of John Farquharson Ltd.

Finally, I get to the real core group—my family. Hey, Mom and Dad, thanks for raising Fred and me on a mixture of Adelle Davis and common sense! Thank you, Tad, for all the cooking, cleaning, child care, and love unselfishly given so I could pursue this goal. And, to Mairead, Charna, and Graham, thank you for being our incentives.

# FOOD TO GROW ON
## A parent's guide to nutrition

By Nancy Van Leuven
Foreword by Michael F. Sussman, M.D.

**For Mairead, Charna, and
Graham**

A Storey Publishing Book
Storey Communications, Inc.
Pownal, VT 05261

Cover and text illustrations by Alison Kolesar
Cover design by Debora M. Haskel
Text design and production by Nancy M. Lamb
Typesetting by Jackson Typesetting, Inc., Jackson, MI

Printed in the United States by Banta Company

Second printing, March 1989

**Library of Congress Cataloging-in-Publication Data**

Van Leuven, Nancy, 1951–
    Food to grow on.

    "A Storey Publishing book."
    Bibliography: p.
    Includes index.
    1. Children—Nutrition. I. Title.
RJ206.V35   1988       613.2'088054       87-42971
ISBN 0-88266-491-3 pbk
ISBN 0-88266-490-5 hc

# FOREWORD

**E**VERY DAY I see caregivers—mothers, some fathers, occasional grandparents and foster parents. Most are in their twenties, some are in their teens, but more and more are in their thirties and early forties. Most are with their first and second child, occasionally their third child, rarely their fourth. Some are on federal support, many work part or full time, some live part of the week in the city and part in my area. Many are single caregivers, by accident, by choice, by convenience, by law.

They all are concerned with the growth, nutrition, and well-being of their children. They express questions, worries, and ideas about growth and nutrition at all points of the children's development—from the newborn's first office visit to the high school physical. Their thoughts have been shaped not only by the way *they* were raised, but also by constant bombardment from the media, their neighbors, friends, relatives—even the milkman. Their needs are so varied!

What can I tell them?

In every area of nutrition and growth there is disagreement, different priorities, varied needs. More and more I find my advice has become broader, less specific: increasingly I want to tell the caregiver to do what she or he thinks is right for the child. *Food to Grow On* offers basic information and advice, and then encourages readers to make their own decisions. The author attempts to demystify and simplify feeding a child. Her light and gentle manner will help parents and other caregivers to relax. I as a pediatrician increasingly find myself echoing her advice to stop complicating the subject, to offer foods that are minimally processed—and that if the child doesn't eat them today, she will eat them tomorrow, and can still go to college!

One message of the book is that it is not more difficult to provide a balanced, less processed diet. This message comes across throughout the book, whether Ms. Van Leuven is discussing the advantages of breastfeeding or methods of coaxing a school system into having a nutrition policy concerning snacks. Experts can disagree about the correlation between test scores and diet, or whether a child given vitamin supplements will come down with fewer colds. But I am sure they are all in agreement with Ms. Van Leuven concerning the importance of presenting food to satisfy the child's nutritional needs, and not "to please Mommy."

I suspect that any of my above patients will find *Food to Grow On* a reassuring and comforting support in their day-to-day decisions on *what* and *why* and *how* to feed their children. I think you will, too. Even if you read the book once and do not return for its recipes, you will have gained in knowledge and self-confidence.

Michael F. Sussman, M.D., F.A.A.P.
Williamstown Medical Associates
Williamstown, Massachusetts

# INTRODUCTION

**A**S PARENTS, one of our greatest and most constant challenges is choosing the healthiest way to feed our families. We need to know how to make good selections from the foods that are available, and then how to put these foods together. This book will guide parents along the way toward feeding their children best through the first seven years of life.

I've focused on simple ways to make nutritious, whole foods attractive. Each chapter corresponds to a stage in your child's development, since nutritional and other needs vary so much in the first years. The recipes are so easy that your child will soon be cooking with you. Together, you will steer your entire family toward a delicious and superior diet of lean meats, less refined foods, and unsaturated foods.

Some topics will pop up repeatedly, such as snacking, cooking with your child, and label reading. These ideas become more complicated as your child grows, and each chapter focuses on new ways for her growing mind to learn about nutrition. Before you know it, your underfoot toddler will be an older child who knows a lot about how to cook and eat what's best for her.

Just as your doctor often picks and chooses between medical studies, you can gather from this book what is best for your family. This is not a medical text, since parents should consult with their doctor about their child's health. You're no doubt aware that every expert or medical study may tell you something different: while one pediatrician will tell you that sugar contributes to hyperactivity, another will refute that claim; while one study will conclude that vitamin supplements aren't needed for children over one year old, another will advise a strict regimen for people of all ages. You will often have to rely on your instincts, as well as those of a doctor with whom you're comfortable.

Finally, I've included charts of quality children's foods and the quantities of them that kids need. Don't feel you must adhere strictly to these guidelines, since kids manage to be happy and healthy despite our worries. As long as we offer an appetizing variety of good foods in a pleasant atmosphere, most kids will eat what they need.

Our common goal is to nurture and nourish our families. While we might choose different paths, we all hope to see the same reward: children with bright, shining eyes, abundant energy, and flourishing health. Offering food to grow on is a wonderful way to achieve that goal.

To your happy, healthy family!

# 1 PRENATAL NUTRITION:
## *A Great Beginning*

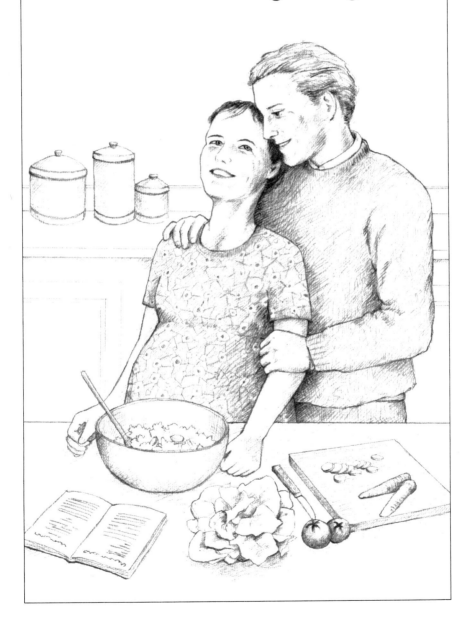

**C**ONGRATULATIONS! YOU'RE going to become parents. Over the next nine months, you'll go through an infinite number of changes to accommodate the new life growing within you. This is a time of questioning everything, from what you want out of life to ways of parenting and goals for nutrition.

You'll want to know all your choices. Read everything you can (see Recommended Readings and Resources at the back of this book) that is helpful and upbeat. You'll find, as we have, that the healthiest and happiest family comes naturally, with whole foods and breastfeeding in the critical early stages.

After much reading, you'll know more about having the easiest pregnancy and delivery. You already know instinctively how to give birth all by yourself, but you need reassurance, support, and the proper tools.

Choose the best doctor available to deliver your baby, one who shares your philosophy of childbirth. This person will literally hold your child's life in his or her hands, and perhaps your own life as well. Your choice is called the Fifth Freedom by the American Medical Association: *your right to select a doctor sympathetic to your needs.*

So don't automatically sign up with your best friend's doctor or the lowest-priced hospital! Shop around for your ideal birth environment. Call your local hospitals and ask for an obstetrical nurse who will describe both the facility and the doctors who deliver there. Consider touring the hospitals that appeal to you most. Ask other parents who delivered their baby, and why they chose him or her. Even if you know in your heart that you have the ideal candidate, be doubly sure you share the same goals.

As the mom of three children born in entirely different situations, I've benefited greatly from interviews with obstetricians and pediatricians long before my due dates. That way, I've known in advance how liberal or conservative my doctors were in such areas as prenatal diet and exercise, natural childbirth, and breastfeeding on demand. Write down and ask questions about the topics that are important to you before you sign a payment contract with any doctor.

And listen carefully for *how* a doctor answers you; even if she's heard your questions a million times before, she should be sympathetic and polite. Will you feel comfortable calling her in the middle of the night, or will you feel apologetic? In short, choose the OB and hospital that will make you feel most at ease.

For instance, one OB I interviewed just nodded and rolled his eyes in exasperation when I asked if our baby could be nursed on demand. I later heard that he routinely orders nurses to give sugar water to all newborns before nursing, a dreadful practice that can work against successful breastfeeding.

In contrast, another doctor gave me stacks of pamphlets about different birthing methods and the superiority of breastmilk. Guess which one delivered our daughter?

# Why Breastfeeding Is Best Feeding

Even before you feel the first flutter of life, your baby has formed nearly all her organs and a foundation for future health. You are initially her sole provider of life-giving food, and what you're feeding her through your diet may determine how many brain cells she's blessed with and whether she'll be a healthy, happy child.

And so it is after birth. The most natural, easy way to feed your baby is with your own body, just as you did when you carried her. More important, breastmilk is superior to formulas, none of which can duplicate its vitamins, antibodies, and immune factors. In trying to copy breastmilk, most formula manufacturers add synthetic vitamins to cow's milk, evaporated milk powder, granulated sugar, corn syrup, and brown sugar.

Cow's milk is best for baby cows: human milk is best for baby humans.

## Your Own Milk's Value Cannot Be Duplicated

This entire book could be filled with scientific data on the superiority of breastmilk. In a nutshell, nursing gives babies the best nutritional well-being and helps form a strong bond between mother and child.

Its immune factors are especially valuable: breastmilk contains substances that prevent the growth of harmful bacteria in the intestinal tract and encourage friendly bacteria. Breastmilk also provides interferon, an anti-viral factor not present in formula, as well as lactose and amino acids especially important in the development of your baby's brain. Because it is so perfectly suited to humans, a baby quickly digests breastmilk without problems, as opposed to some foreign milk sources.

The difference between a bottlefed and breastfed baby goes beyond what's in his stomach. Many doctors and pediatric dentists feel that a nursing baby's sucking activity provides good tongue thrust and jaw development. And a nursing baby just looks and feels wonderful. Fueled naturally, his skin is soft, he smells sweet, and his breath is angelic. Even his dirty diapers smell better.

Finally, breastfeeding is invaluable for a mother who nurses immediately following delivery since it activates two hormones, oxytocin and prolactin. Oxytocin helps expel the placenta, shrinks the uterus back to its normal size, pushes out the placenta, and helps reduce bleeding. Prolactin is a "loving" hormone with such maternal power that if it's injected into a rooster, it causes him to mother tiny chicks.

The American Academy of Pediatrics recommends that you nurse your baby for at least one year, with breastmilk alone for the first six months. For more information, ask your doctor, *and* call your local La Leche League chapter.


**Food for Thought.** *Colostrum* is the yellowish liquid your nursing baby receives during the first few days of life. What a gold mine it is, packed with just the right amount of protein, minerals, sugar, and fat for a newborn. Studies have shown that colostrum contains at least five times as much protein as breastmilk, yet only half the carbohydrates. In addition, while a baby receives some antibodies through the placenta *in utero*, colostrum doubles that amount. Its antibody content (which protect your infant from infection) is at its peak during the first twelve hours after birth. Colostrum acts as a laxative for your baby's first bowel movement of sticky, black meconium. Even if you don't plan to nurse for long, give your baby an initial gift of this precious food. ∎

Toward the end of your pregnancy, you may see a bit of colostrum on your nipples. Your breasts are already preparing themselves for their natural function: nourishing your newborn.

## Prenatal Nipple Care

I've found it helpful to toughen my nipples during the last month of pregnancy. Other moms agree that simply leaving off their bra or gently rubbing their nipples with a washcloth is beneficial.

You can also condition your nipples by pulling them out firmly, though never painfully. It's a good idea to buy some pure lanolin to rub in toward the end of your pregnancy (unless you're allergic to wool), and again if your nipples become tender during the first weeks of nursing.

To help prevent engorgement when your milk comes in, you can hand-express some colostrum to open your milk ducts. Use the same method as when you express milk later on (see the next chapter for tips on draining your milk reservoirs).

Many pregnant moms follow a routine of expressing colostrum and conditioning their nipples twice a day for the last six weeks of pregnancy. This treatment is especially helpful for women with inverted nipples, which can be gently drawn out before delivery. Try to follow a schedule, such as during your morning shower and at night when you undress.

Don't use soap on your nipples while you're pregnant or nursing. It acts as a drying agent and can cause cracking. Just wash with plain water.

## Last Words About Old Wives' Tales

As a La Leche League leader, I've talked with hundreds of women about the joys and pitfalls of breastfeeding. And I am constantly amazed at the rumors and fears that keep some mothers from enjoying their womanly instincts. For example:

**Breast size** has nothing to do with whether you can nurse. Some of the smallest breasts literally drip with milk. One overproducing mom asked me where all her milk ducts were hiding, since they certainly weren't, as she put it, "above board"! Large-breasted women can enjoy equal success. Your baby doesn't care about the size of your breast, only that you have a nipple.

**Modesty** is frequently a concern of would-be nursers. While some moms feel they could never nurse in front of anybody, others nurse everywhere, from the mall to the church. Their secret is discretion, which depends in large part on their clothing. Plan now on wearing half-slips and two-piece outfits. You can easily pull up your top, and your baby will cover the rest of you.

**Time** is on your side when you breastfeed. Somebody needs to feed the baby anyway, so wouldn't you rather be the one to put up your feet and give him the best? Nursing saves you from fussing with bottles and formula. Your breastmilk is warm, sterile, antibiotic, nutritious, and convenient. It also saves you a great deal of money.

Think about it. Besides being nutritionally superior for your baby, breastfeeding is best for you as well. There is nothing so refreshing and renewing as sitting down to nurse your baby. While the following chapter gives specific "how-to's," for now simply say to yourself, "I can!"

# Needs and Priorities: Putting Baby First

You can lay the foundation for a great pregnancy and baby *before* you become pregnant. Once you have a child growing within you, those nine months give him the basic constitution he will carry the rest of his life.

Even in its first two weeks (usually before your pregnancy test!), your fetus depends on the nutrients already stored in your body. And during the first three months of pregnancy, your diet is especially crucial to the health of your baby's tissues and organs and to the life-giving placenta.

Dad should eat a healthy diet of whole foods, too. A man's diet affects everything from his sperm count to his energy levels. Give yourselves a well-rounded diet so that the entire family will be better prepared for labor, birth, and the responsibilities of caring for a new baby.

Literally *everything* you eat, drink, and breathe can reach your baby and affect its development. Heaven knows we have enough worries already about "Will our baby be healthy?" to give ourselves any reason to feel guilty later. Read labels and trust your instincts: you'll naturally turn to food to grow on.

> **The statistics are undeniable: alcohol can kill brain cells. Smoking can cause cancer. And both can result in smaller, more sickly, and more malformed**

**babies than if their Mom abstained. In one test reported by the American Cancer Society, seven-year-old children of heavy smokers were shorter and had lower reading and social skills than children of non-smoking mothers.**

Warnings are everywhere, from cigarette to cold-capsule packages. A recent ordinance passed in Los Angeles County requires signs everywhere liquor is sold, including restaurants, noting that alcohol can cause birth defects.

So whether you're tempted by junk food, caffeine, cigarettes, drugs, or alcohol, think of pregnancy as nine months of Lent. And remember, it won't be long before your child will be imitating you. What a great reason to keep up the good work!

## Back to Basics

Whether you're feeding an embryo or a family of eight, a well-balanced diet should include several servings from each of the food groups. Have three small meals and lots of nutritious snacks throughout the day. Your expanding uterus may not leave much room for huge meals, and snacks help ward off morning sickness and heartburn. Such "grazing" keeps up our blood sugar and is better for all of us. Settle into the habit now, and keep it throughout your nursing and long afterward.

Ask your doctor about the best prenatal diet for you. In addition to prescribing extra vitamins and iron, he'll advise you on calorie intake and the types of food you need.

Eat lots of fresh vegetables while you are pregnant, especially those with dark green leaves. Also ask your doctor about taking extra folic acid (your need has doubled), iron (take with vitamin C to help its absorption), and calcium with magnesium, especially during the last half of pregnancy when your baby may rob your bones to make his own.

**For a simple source of calcium, try adding a teaspoon of *blackstrap molasses* into a glass of milk. The milk's calcium content will be increased by more than ten percent!**

## For the Best-Built Baby, Pregnant and Nursing Women Can Eat:

**Protein**, 3 servings daily, such as: 3 ounces lean meat, fish, or poultry; ½ cup tuna fish; 2 eggs; 1 cup cooked dried lentils, beans, or peas; or 4 tablespoons peanut butter.

**Milk and dairy products**, 4 servings daily, such as: 1 cup of milk, yogurt, custard or milk pudding; 1½ cups cottage cheese; 1½ ounces natural cheese. Vary your sources of dairy foods—some babies get milk allergies if their moms drink too much milk during pregnancy. For example, eat ½ pound of cottage cheese or ¼ pound of cheese to equal one pint of milk. Or take calcium and magnesium, and ask your doctor about other milk substitutes.

**Fruits and vegetables,** 4 servings including a daily vitamin C source. Try for at least one raw salad a day. ½ cup equals one serving.

**Whole grain breads and cereals**, at least 6 servings, such as: whole slice of bread; ½ cup cooked cereal, rice, or noodles; or ¾ cup dry cereal.

You'll need about thirty percent more vitamins and protein than before you were pregnant, as well as a hefty increase in water. Drink several tall glasses of water a day to flush out your system and avoid constipation. After birth, you'll keep on drinking that amount to make breastmilk.

## The Weighting Game

Although the old concept of "eating for two" has been buried, you are still the sole provider for your baby. Nowadays, few doctors call for a rigid "don't gain over twenty pounds" mandate. This is because a direct link has been shown between a mother's weight gain and that of her baby.

Just as some women have big babies, they also have varying weight increases. Some gain as much as forty pounds during pregnancy, and then shed it (nursing helps) soon after birth. Others live in deadly fear of the doctor's scales and actually diet during pregnancy, which can malnourish a baby!

You'll probably gain about twenty pounds by the time you're five months pregnant, then about two pounds per month until delivery. How much you gain isn't as important as when you gain, since excessive, sudden weight gain can be a warning signal.

**A surprising weight spurt might be a symptom of toxemia during pregnancy, a fairly common complication which is often prevented by a good prenatal diet. Your physician's routine tests (urine, weight check, and blood pressure) will pick up many symptoms, and you should report any severe persistent headache, fever, dizziness, or abdominal pain. Most doctors advise toxemia patients to put up their feet, cut down on sodium, and get lots of bed rest.**

Personally, I gain a lot of weight during pregnancy, especially during my last month. While the doctor who delivered our first baby was unconcerned, the OB for our second child immediately suggested that I go on a strict diet. But all that extra weight had a definite purpose: it went straight to our daughter, who weighed in at nearly ten pounds! I was glad that I listened to my instincts.

## Where Your Extra Weight Goes:

7½ pounds . . . . . . . . average weight of baby
4 pounds . . . . . . . . . . increased volume of blood
6 to 10 pounds . . . . . increased fluid retention and maternal fat stores
2 pounds . . . . . . . . . . placental fluid
1½ pounds . . . . . . . . increased weight of breasts
1½ pounds . . . . . . . . placenta
2 pounds . . . . . . . . . increased weight in expanded uterus

**About 30 pounds expected gain during pregnancy**

As long as you're eating whole foods, don't worry about your weight unless your doctor does. Even an overweight woman shouldn't consume less than 2,000 calories per day. You should consume about fifteen percent *more* calories for your increased energy needs. You need enough dietary fat, for instance, to make use of the protein you eat, so that it goes directly into building your baby's body. Your happy attitude during pregnancy shouldn't be dampened by worry over pounds you'll later lose.

The only good reason for actually counting calories might be because you're gaining excessive weight from *empty* calories or too much fat. Think of calories as the energy in your food that you burn up as you go about your daily activities. Before your pregnancy, you'd gain a pound if you ate 3,600 more calories than you used up.

So try to make calories count. Table sugar, for example, fills you with empty calories that can stimulate your appetite and cause you to eat more than you need. It is a simple carbohydrate that gives calories with little nutritive value in the way of vitamins, minerals, or protein. Yet it goes into your blood stream and can cause your blood sugar level to skyrocket, then crash, leaving you with nothing but a crabby mood, extra calories, and a craving for more sweets.

Be careful of excessive fats, as well. Over consumption of saturated fats, such as butter, animal fats, and coconut and peanut oils, has been implicated in heart and blood vessel disease.

To trim fat from your diet:
- Use lemon juice on your salads rather than oil-based, fatty salad dressings.
- Season with spices and herbs rather than butter or sauces.
- Use oil instead of shortening.
- Stir-fry your vegetables in a dab of oil.
- Lightly steam, broil, or bake your foods.
- De-fat your foods by substituting cottage cheese or skinned chicken for beef.
- Exercise: take a 45-minute brisk walk four times a week, and you'll lose twenty pounds a year without dieting!

Instead of cooking with highly saturated products such as bacon drippings and shortening, use unsaturated fats such as vegetable and fish oils. These are thought to be less likely to plug up arteries, and they'll help keep your weight down.

## Natural Cures For Common Complaints

**Constipation** is unfortunately a common problem, even among non-pregnant people. Indeed, the amount of laxatives now sold is incredible. Use natural remedies, such as increased fiber and liquids. Besides relieving constipation and reducing your appetite, fibers in fruits and vegetables act like a sponge in your intestinal tract as they soak up and remove extra substances. The best sources of fiber are whole grains, bran, fruit (dried, stewed, or raw) and vegetables. Walking helps your digestive system, and is a healthy cure. And elevate your feet with a footstool when you're on the toilet. Ask your doctor if the type of iron in your prenatal vitamin could be contributing to your constipation. Some health food stores carry natural, chelated iron supplements that don't affect the bowels.

**Frequent urination**, like constipation, will lessen after the first trimester and return the last three months. It's caused by your enlarging uterus pressing on your bladder, so the only remedy is your sense of humor and a lot of Kegel exercises (contract or tighten your pelvic muscles as if to stop urinating). Continue to drink three quarts of liquid a day so that you won't get a kidney or bladder infection. Getting up so many times in the night may actually be nature's way of preparing you for getting up with your baby!

**Food for Thought.** Many remedies are cheap, natural, and more effective than their drugstore counterparts. I've found a neck massage and a large glass of water usually gets rid of a headache faster than any aspirin. And kids love a cough syrup of warm honey and lemon juice. *Herbs* are especially wonderful during pregnancy and just after birth when your cells are changing so rapidly. For instance, use comfrey in your bath to reduce swelling, and enjoy relaxing red raspberry tea throughout your pregnancy. For a free pamphlet, send a self-addressed, stamped legal-size envelope for "Natural Remedies for Pregnancy Discomforts" to the Department of Consumer Affairs, P.O. Box 310, Sacramento, CA, 95802. ■

**Morning sickness** may be caused by hormonal changes during your first trimester. Many doctors feel that nausea or vomiting can be caused by a low level of vitamin $B_6$, which your liver needs to cope with extra female hormones. Don't take any medication without your doctor's approval. Your natural solution: frequent protein snacks, such as nuts, cheese, and other foods high in B complex vitamins. To guard against low blood sugar, eat some protein foods just before bedtime and as soon as you get up. Throughout the first three months of my pregnancies, I snacked at least every two hours, with great results. If food odors bother you, turn on fans and open windows to get rid of them.

**Fatigue** is another common symptom during the first and last trimesters. Think of it as the baby trying to get you to rest so he can grow. Try to get up on schedule, take naps, and go to bed early. I sometimes think our early-pregnancy sleeping is a way of storing up for the insomnia of the last month, when an active baby, frequent urination, and false labor make sleep next to impossible. Get creative with pillow placement, and use the time to read more about parenting!

**Other aches and pains** include upper backaches, which are helped by overhead reaches, head and shoulder circles, and good posture. Lower backaches respond to frequent pelvic rocks and roll-backs on the floor. Heartburn is caused by your stomach being crowded; drink water and eat small meals. Women with leg cramps find relief with increased calcium, vitamin E, and leg rubs. For headaches, massage your shoulders, temples, and the base of your skull. Any sharp pains in your groin area come from the stretching of the round ligaments that support your growing uterus. Before coughing and sneezing, be sure to draw your knees up a bit, and avoid sudden twists at the waist. Also try some exercises on-the-job: walk around at least every hour (in place, if necessary), put up your feet when possible, and stretch out your arms, shoulders, back, and neck.

Prompt, early medical attention can help solve the most serious complications of pregnancy. If your pregnancy isn't trouble free, take it from me: it will be much more tolerable if you keep your sense of humor and love. The most we can do is give our babies the best chance for good health.

## • Warning Signs •
*Call your doctor at once if you have*
*any of these problems during pregnancy:*

- Sudden swelling or puffiness of the eyes, fingers, or face

- Blurred vision

- Unrelenting severe headaches

- Bright red vaginal bleeding

- Severe, persistent pain in your abdomen

- Water bag breakage (rupture of the membrane causing water seepage)

- Sudden lack of fetal movement over a twenty-four-hour period

- Fever

- Persistent vomiting

- Major decrease in amount of urination

## The Extra Protection of Supplements

Not so long ago, people didn't take extra vitamins. Their food was grown with natural fertilizers in good soil, free of modern chemicals, sprays, and polluted air and water. Today I feel we *must* use supplements because we can't be sure our food is whole and pure. Natural vitamins, free of artificial additives and sugar, can make up for many deficiencies in our food sources.

Supplements are especially advisable during pregnancy, when both mother and baby are preparing for birth. Ask your doctor what she recommends. Teamed with a superior diet, supplements can give you extra stamina for a superior pregnancy. And a well-nourished fetus will have optimal health and the maximum growth of brain cells.

The following chart shows some foods especially high in certain nutrients. I find this kind of information even more valuable when my children go through picky stages. If they seem stressed and I want to increase their Vitamin $B_6$ intake, for example, I slip wheat germ into their cooked cereal, or fix egg salad sandwiches. Before I nag them to eat all their lovely green spinach, I hand them some other iron-rich food, such as bananas or raisins. Pregnant moms should follow the same idea. After all, it's not important which foods give us our nourishment, just that they do one way or another, in a diet that's as pure, varied, and delicious as possible.

## WHAT NUTRIENTS DO, AND SOME NATURAL SOURCES

| Vitamin | What it does | Where it's found |
|---|---|---|
| Vitamin A | Maintains healthy skin, improves vision, fights infection | Green leafy vegetables<br>Carrots, cantaloupe<br>Yellow vegetables<br>Tomatoes<br>Liver, egg yolk<br>Cod liver oil |
| $B_1$, Thiamine | Good for growth, teeth, gums<br>Helps carbohydrate metabolism<br>Stimulates appetite | Meats<br>Vegetables<br>Whole grains<br>Brewer's yeast |
| $B_2$, Riboflavin | Deficiency causes hair loss, burning of eyes, tongue, lips | Found in the same foods as thiamine |
| Niacin | Deficiency causes pellagra, reddening of body parts, nerve problems, and stomach upsets | Found in the same foods as thiamine |

| | | |
|---|---|---|
| B<sub>6</sub>, Pyridoxine | Helps digest fats<br>Makes healthy blood | Egg yolk<br>Wheat germ<br>Yeast |
| $B_{12}$ | Treats certain blood disorders | Liver, meats, fish<br>sea vegetables,<br>fermented foods |
| Vitamin C,<br>Ascorbic Acid | Prevents colds and infections<br>Makes gums, teeth, joints<br>healthy | Potatoes<br>Fruits<br>Citrus<br>Raw green foods |
| Vitamin D | Makes strong bones and teeth | Sunshine<br>Cod liver oil<br>Kidneys, liver<br>Oysters |
| Vitamin E | Protects blood<br>Helps skin heal | Green vegetables<br>Wheat germ oil |
| Vitamin K | Prevents hemorrhaging | Made in intestines |
| Calcium | Strengthens bones, teeth,<br>muscles, nerve function | Dairy products,<br>wheat germ, nuts,<br>sardines, beans<br>and legumes,<br>cabbage, turnip<br>greens, kale,<br>other green<br>vegetables,<br>blackstrap molasses |
| Iron | Prevents anemia; vital in<br>production of red blood<br>cells | Seeds, eggs, raisins, beans,<br>green leafy vegetables,<br>meat, fish, brewer's<br>yeast, wheat germ,<br>almonds, parsley,<br>prunes |
| Potassium | Helps in cell function<br>Prevents weak muscles | Nuts<br>Fruits<br>Seeds |
| Zinc | Essential for good skin,<br>growth, wound healing | Seafood<br>Kelp<br>Rarely found in<br>processed foods |

Listen to your cravings. If you're downing lots of oranges, chances are your body is craving the nutrients oranges provide. When you reach for a candy bar, ask yourself if you're really after a quick sugar fix that you could be getting from fruit!

As you continue to read more about whole foods, you'll find more information about how vitamin and mineral supplements can be remedies for everything from sleep problems to hyperactivity. I especially recommend the books in "Recommended Readings and Resources," and encourage you to ask your doctor for other ideas.

# Creating A Diet of Foods to Grow On

Building a strong baby is simple if you keep in mind some basic nutritional concepts such as food groups and vitamins. By starting healthy meal plans now, you'll be accustomed to eating superior food when your baby grabs for her first bites. Pregnancy is a great reason to start a lifelong habit of good nutrition.

The following guidelines come from many interviews with doctors, nutritionists, educators, and families. As with all advice, take it at your own speed. Just as some smokers prefer to quit slowly instead of cold turkey, you may prefer to ease into a lifestyle of better food rather than jumping in all at once.

## Easing Away From Refined Foods

First, take stock of how many refined foods you're eating. White flour and sugar, for instance, have snuck their way into our diets without many of us realizing just how ever-present and worthless they are. Giving your body such empty foods is like going to work all day and not getting paid for it.

Read labels to find out if the ingredients in your favorite foods are natural or synthetic. Many packaged foods contain more than their labels imply. Canned corn, for instance, usually contains corn syrup or sugar. And the amount of additives, colorings, and preservatives in processed and packaged foods seems boundless.

Food manufacturers and supermarket owners seem to favor chemicals which enable food to last indefinitely. Unfortunately, consumers have grown to expect the taste and convenience these chemicals have made possible, especially since processed food is sometimes less expensive than its natural counterparts.

**For instance, you'll spend more for a no-salt can of soup than a salted one. Companies defend the higher cost by saying that salt-free soup needs more natural herbs and spices for taste. In other words, we have to pay more to enjoy natural goodness!**

Now, while you're waiting for the birth of your baby, take some time to discover the joys of cooking from scratch. You'll find recipes and support at places besides the supermarket. The people of your local whole foods store, for instance, can help start you on a more natural diet.

## The Goodness of Grains

*Grains* are a core of complete meals. When combined with nuts, dairy products, or beans and peas, the amount of usable protein is much higher than if we ate each food separately. Try to use *whole* grains instead of refined ones, which are stripped of their nutrient-rich outer layers and their germ.

It's not always easy to switch from the light, fluffy textures of white, refined rice and flour to the nutty, heavier textures of whole grains. If you do use white flour, try using half unbleached white and half whole wheat flour in your recipes. Make a gradual transition until your food contains only the whole, complete wheat flour, which has nearly four times more fiber than white flour.

Do try making your own bread! Even the most hard-core, bleached flour fanatic adores home-baked bread made from whole wheat flour. I've included a few very easy recipes in this book, including a slow-cooker version.

Here is a mini-encyclopedia of grains that may help you progress beyond the usual white bread/white rice emphasis of our national diet:

# A GUIDE TO WHOLE GRAINS

**AMARANTH.** A rich source of protein, calcium, and other nutrients.

**BARLEY.** Used in beer brewing. Add to your bread and rice.

**BRAN.** Husks of grains, sifted from the flour and partly ground.

**BUCKWHEAT.** Use it in bread, porridge, pancakes, and dumplings.

**BULGUR.** Parboiled and cracked wheat, popular in Middle Eastern dishes. Can replace cracked wheat in many recipes.

**CORN.** Buy stoneground, whole grain cornmeal rather than degerminated. Wonderful as a vegetable or ground and used in breads, mush, and tortillas.

**CRACKED WHEAT.** Broken grains, delicious when used as rice or cooked as cereal. Make your own by whirling some whole wheat berries in your blender, then sifting out the flour.

**GERM.** The living part of the grain, the embryo of the cereal plant containing much of its vitamins, minerals, and oil.

**GROATS.** Whole kernels that have been cleaned, toasted, hulled, and scoured.

**MILLET.** A tiny yellow grain that can be steamed like rice or stirred to eat as porridge or in place of mashed potatoes.

**OATS.** Contain twice as much protein as corn or wheat; also iron, calcium, and seven other minerals, as well as seven B vitamins and vitamin E. Make your own oat flour by grinding rolled oats in a blender or food processor (blend with other whole grain flours so that your baked goods will rise). One cup oats makes ¾ cup oat flour.

**RICE.** The dietary staple of over half the world's people. Can be ground and used with other flours for light-baked goods.

**ROLLED OATS.** Old-fashioned method is to flatten and steam whole groats with a roller. Avoid instant oats, since they are pre-cooked and nearly always contain salt and sugar.

**RYE.** Makes a filling, dark, heavy loaf, a nice change from wheat breads.

**SORGHUM.** One of the most popular grains in Asia and Africa, some varieties are grown as a source of sweet syrups. Can be used as rice or ground into meal for baked goods.

**TRITICALE.** A cross between wheat and rye.

**WHEAT BERRIES.** Hulled kernels.

**WHOLE WHEAT FLOUR.** Available in regular texture or pastry, which is finely sifted. Buy stone ground flour to avoid the rancid oil in flour ground with a high-speed roller mill. Or buy wheat berries and grind your own!

---

It's fascinating to learn how whole grains have dominated the diets and maintained the health of traditional cultures. For instance, Latin dishes combine rice, corn, and beans to supply ample quantities of protein, while many Chinese recipes combine rice and soybeans (tofu). Those peoples whose diets are based on whole grains have markedly fewer bowel and intestinal illnesses, thanks to the vitamins, minerals, and fibers of unrefined foods. Our modern Western society, on the other hand, bases its diet on dairy products, meat, and refined instead of whole grains.

Try making your next lasagna with spinach instead of ground beef. You'll save money, improve your family's health, and discover a delicious new meatless dish.

## Moving Away from Meat

Our society is meat-crazy. Actually, we're protein-crazy, since most of us eat two to five times more protein than we need. And, according to *Jane Brody's Nutrition Book*, at least seventy percent of Americans' protein comes from eating animal foods. It's an expensive way to absorb cholesterol and fat.

And our meat sources are far from pure. Some beef and poultry growers sterilize and pacify their animals with antibiotics and other drugs. Many of these chemicals remain in body tissues, which means we can end up eating hormones, tenderizers, and dyes. A pregnant woman (and growing children) should be especially wary of processed meats such as bacon, frankfurters, and ham if they contain the suspected carcinogens nitrates and nitrites.

**Food for Thought.** Many adults and children thrive on vegetarian diets. To reduce your meat intake gradually, serve a meatless dish every other day and cut out red meat while continuing to eat fish, turkey, and chicken. Perhaps you'll eventually eat meat once a week or less. However, a few vegetarian diets might not be suitable for children or women who are pregnant or lactating unless they add extra supplements. For instance, a child's vegan diet without meat, eggs, or milk products might lack calcium, zinc, riboflavin, and vitamin $B_{12}$. A fruitarian diet of fruits and nuts could be deficient in protein, while a macrobiotic diet followed carelessly might lack protein and vitamin $B_{12}$. A diet of raw foods may not contain enough carbohydrates for growing children. Like all diets, a vegetarian approach should include a variety of foods, and can easily be balanced by using cooked vegetables, raw fruit, legumes (peas and beans), seeds and nuts, and fermented foods. Such a diet is perfectly healthy and natural. ■

> **The bottom line: if you eat meat, be careful about where it comes from, what non-meat ingredients are included in it, and whether it's properly cleaned and cooked. Don't ever eat undercooked chicken, and don't transfer bacteria from raw meat to other foods by using the same knife or cutting board without cleaning them first.**

Thanks to consumer requests, a number of supermarkets now carry frozen hot dogs and sausages without sugar and nitrites. But store owners won't stock healthy food to grow on unless they are sure that you'll buy it, so let them know that you want unrefined foods and pure meat and produce.

It's amazing how one remark can create an avalanche of results. For instance, a chance suggestion by Frank Scalzo (a buyer for the Mrs. Gooch's chain of health food stores) led to a new line of Gran'ma's House sliced luncheon meats. Finally, we can eat a sandwich with pure, additive-free meat! How many more companies would offer better products if they knew we wanted them?

## Fruits and Veggies: Eating Seasonally

Another principle of good nutrition is to eat produce only when it's in season. Apples, for instance, are best eaten during their harvest times, beginning in May and peaking in November. Otherwise, the crunchy russets have been in cold storage and possibly treated with preservatives.

The same is true for bright-red tomatoes, which are usually picked long before you buy them at a supermarket. To survive their long journey, most tomatoes are picked while hard and green, then artificially reddened with ethylene gas. Vine-ripened tomatoes, on the other hand, are flavorful at room temperature and carry a lot more Vitamin C.

If you want to taste delicious summer fruits next winter, can them yourself in honey syrup, or freeze an unsweetened batch of berries or strawberries. Farmer's markets are great places to buy the freshest in-season produce possible.

**One economical parent makes a wonderful soup on her weekly bread-baking day. She saves her family's leftover vegetables in a large freezer bowl and then simmers them in a pot of water for stock. About half an hour before dinner, she strains the stock, puts it back on the stove with fresh vegetables and seasonings, and serves along with freshly baked bread. The two smells are unbeatable together, and everybody loves to eat these vegetables!**

Some final tips on improving your produce: if you use sprayed fruits or vegetables, wash them carefully with a little bit of pure soap and a vegetable scrubber. To retain as many vitamins as possible, don't peel anything except for those highly-waxed apples and cucumbers that are chemical traps. You may find yourself eating a lot more carrots and potatoes once you stop making yourself peel them!

# Sharing Costs: Food Clubs and Co-ops

Unfortunately, healthier foods in some areas are often more expensive. But no matter what type of food you prefer, you'll save money if you join or start a bulk buying group with some of your like-minded friends. A food club is usually run by one person who earns a profit, while a co-op requires all its members to share in management. Either way, participants pay less than retail for their food.

There is probably already a group in your area. Many Mormon churches operate food clubs for items such as whole grains, peanut butter, and cheese. You can also look in your phone book for wholesale health foods distributors and ask if they serve a local co-op.

If not, how about starting your own? Ask local food outlets (such as produce markets, dairies, health food wholesalers, nut and grain dealers) if they deliver to non-storefront customers who can meet their minimum order requirements.

**Local dairies offer cheese and powdered milk in bulk. Nut butters, nuts, and dried fruits are much cheaper when discounted by nut-packing plants. Grain mills sell bags of whole grains and legumes, often packaged for long storage and marked at a fraction of supermarket prices. Bakeries often give fifty-percent price reductions to buyers of large quantities. Also check with your local farmers markets for seasonal produce. Although a bag of oranges typically sells for one dollar, we buy 25-pound crates for four dollars!**

Co-op members can meet once a month (a park is perfect if you have children) to tally their order. Members can talk among themselves about who might want to split ten pounds of pasta or a case of tomato soup. Or several friends can order and later divide a fifteen-pound block of cheese, usually saving at least a dollar per pound.

On the other hand, managing a food club is a great part-time job for a parent who wants to work at home. You can grow as big as you want, depending on how many friends you include on your mailing list (word of mouth travels very fast) and how many distributors you want to deal with.

See Appendix A, page 226: "How to Run a Food Club."

## Supermarket Survival Tips

Food clubs and co-ops provide exciting ways to save money and meet new friends. You can also save money simply by altering your shopping habits. Buying in bulk is one of the easiest ways to reduce your food bills and improve your diet. For instance, you get identical protein from either dried or canned beans, yet dried beans cost less than half what canned beans do. By cooking dried beans according to your favorite recipes, you'll more than double your money.

Some other defensive maneuvers for you to employ in our modern supermarkets, which tempt us with over 15,000 items:

- Prepare a list for about a week's worth of staples.

- Don't shop while you're hungry.

- Buy only the items you've listed.

- Be wary of high-profit convenience foods (usually with zero nutrition) that grocers display at checkout counters and low eye-levels to entice kids.

- Take your children shopping! They need to develop good manners (such as not whining or throwing fits), as well as a familiarity with the healthier items in the store. Our kids especially love to read the labels on canned goods ("What's all this stuff in the juice, Mom?") and packaged meats ("What are all these funny ingredients in this crab?")

Soon enough, your kids will be on their own in the maze of good and not-so-good foods, and it's up to us to teach them ahead of time which path to choose.

# FOOD TO GROW ON SHOPPING LIST:

**Staples**

Baking powder, without aluminum
Baking soda
Baking yeast
Baking mixes, whole grain
Beans, dried
Carob powder
Catsup, unsweetened
Cereals
Cooking Oil, preferably cold-pressed
Cornmeal, whole grain
Crackers
Dried fruits, unsweetened
Eggs, preferably fertile
Flavoring extracts, natural
Flour, whole wheat regular, pastry
Flour, other whole grains
Honey, raw
Jam, unsweetened
Maple syrup, pure Canadian
Mayonnaise, honey or unsweetened
Meat, pure
Molasses
Mustard
Nut butter, natural
Nuts
Oatmeal, non-instant
Pancake mix, whole grain
Pasta
Peas, dried
Pet food
Rice, brown
Salad dressing, pure
Salsa, natural
Seasonings, natural
Seeds, sesame and sunflower
Spaghetti sauce, natural
Tea, herbal
Vinegar
Yeast, baking
Yeast, nutritional

**In-Season Produce:**

Apples
Avocados
Bananas
Beans
Broccoli
Brussels sprouts
Cabbage
Cantaloupe
Carrots
Celery
Corn
Cucumbers
Garlic
Grapefruit
Grapes
Lemons
Lettuce
Onions
Oranges
Peaches
Pears
Peas
Peppers
Pineapple
Plums
Potatoes
Spinach
Strawberries
Tomatoes
Zucchini

**Whole Grain Baked Goods**

Breads
Cakes
Cookies
Rolls, buns

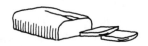

### Canned Goods

Applesauce, unsweetened
Chili, natural
Fruit, unsweetened
Juice, unsweetened
Pumpkin
Soups, natural
Tomato sauce, natural
Tuna, packed in water

### Dairy Products

Butter
Cheese
Frozen yogurt
Ice cream, honey- or
   fruit juice-sweetened
Milk
Sour cream
Yogurt

### Pure Meats

Beef
Chicken
Fish, seafood
Ground meats
Lamb
Liver
Pork
Turkey
Veal

---

# Food for Thought.

If your friends are planning to honor you with a baby shower, suggest some unusual gifts to celebrate your baby's birth. One of our friends held a "Baby Shower on a Shoestring" for us before the birth of our second daughter, and friends brought an assortment of favorite casseroles (with recipes attached) that we could freeze and eat later. Another shower could be for more "personal" gifts, such as parenting magazine subscriptions, gift certificates to natural foods restaurants, or "promise coupons" for a free housecleaning after the baby comes. You'll soon appreciate such tokens much more than yet another yellow and green baby blanket. ■

# FUN IN THE KITCHEN

*Short on time or energy? Try these quick-
as-a-wink protein pick-ups: (Someday,
you'll be fixing these with your child!)*

- Top a scoop of cottage cheese with a dribble of honey or a handful of raisins or blueberries.

- Cream cheese goodies: Roll a bit into a ball, cover it with walnuts, or stuff a date half with cream cheese.

- Make your own GORP (Good Old Raisins and Peanuts). Mix any combination of nuts, dried fruit, and seeds. Some favorites are peanuts, walnuts, raisins, and shelled sunflower seeds.

- Yogurt with a plus: Mix some GORP or wheat germ and fruit into your yogurt for a crunchy breakfast or complete protein snack.

- Orange Potatoes: Cut up a potato and carrot and steam or boil them together until tender. Mash them together and serve with a dab of butter.

- Vary your P.B. and J.: On whole grain bread, try peanut butter with cheese, banana, apple, honey, or wheat germ.

- Ye Olde Grilled Cheese: Add a tomato slice and extra cheese.

- Scrambled eggs: Before they become firm while cooking, add grated cheese, chopped vegetables, onions, sour cream, or whatever you like.

- Frozen vegetables: When you don't have fresh veggies, pop the frozen kind in a covered dish, dab them with butter, and bake alongside your meat or potato at 350° for fifteen minutes or so. A real energy saver!

# 2 NEW MOM AND NEWBORN:
## *The Best Start*

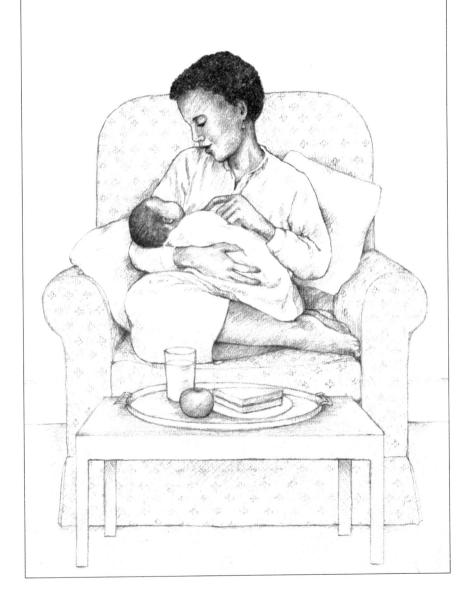

## Between Birth and Six Months, Your Child May

- hold up her head
- turn towards voices
- smile and laugh out loud
- play with her hands and feet
- fit into your family!

**H**URRAH! YOUR wait has ended and your newborn baby is finally here. Could you be any happier or more in love than when your soft, warm baby closes her tiny fingers over yours? Or when her eyes, blinking in a sudden rush of light, catch sight of your face?

Watch her body relax as you caress her, and her tiny rosebud mouth pucker in anticipation of nursing. Her first fumbling attempts may be as comical as they are frustrating: one of our daughters latched right onto the breast within seconds, while the other angrily tried to suck on my nightgown. Our son would dive for fingers, chin, or any other warm possibility.

**Whether you nurse your baby or not, try to have as much physical contact with her as possible right after birth. Research by Dr. Michael Daley has shown that "early contact" babies (who stay with their mothers at least forty-five minutes in the two hours after birth) usually gain weight and eat better, speak earlier, and show a greater vocabulary by the time they are two years old.**

The most successful breastfeeding stories come from less complex cultures where women simply put their baby to breast. Unless you're faced with a medical emergency, your baby belongs with you as much as possible.

Be polite, but ask for your baby! Your milk glands are already working, and you need your baby to suck. The more she sucks, the better your milk supply will be. She needs your warmth, your comforting voices, and your nourishment.

Your mate and you have the right to form a close, spiritual attachment to your newborn. After all, such bonds can affect your family forever.

## Getting the Best Start in The Hospital

- Be firm in your desire for complete rooming-in. If you're told that the hospital is too crowded, ask to be put on a waiting list, and then call to check-up on the list every day.

- Note on your baby's chart if he is to be totally breastfed so that he won't get any bottles without your knowledge. Total breastfeeding will also avoid "nipple confusion" between your nipple and the rigid rubber nipple of a bottle. Since babies use more muscles and effort to nurse than drink from a bottle, some may become too lazy to breastfeed unless you get them used to nursing right away. And you don't want any of your milk to be replaced by formula or water.

- Quietly keep your baby at your breast. Get him interested by simply brushing your nipple across his cheek, and he'll root towards you. (This technique also works for placid babies who want to sleep more than nurse.) Your hospital might have a standard feeding schedule, yet your baby may need more time than the schedule allows. When asked, simply say that he's not done eating yet. Be polite but firm!

- Keep up your vitamins and superior diet. Your baby still depends on you. Drink lots of water, about three quarts of fluid each day if you can.

- Relax and breathe deeply. A baby is very quick to mirror the mood of his parents, so try to make feeding times as peaceful as possible. For instance, grab a glass of water, book, and whatever else you need before you settle down to nurse. Both your baby and you will be much more relaxed.

- Rely on your spouse, family, physician, and others for encouragement and support. Being a parent may not seem natural and easy at first, and you might need encouragement for the first month or so. Don't despair!

# Breastfeeding Tips
# From the First Moment On

Just after delivery, your breasts will automatically adapt to the needs of your newborn. Your nursing baby gets two or three days of precious colostrum before your milk comes in; the combination of the two will at first make your milk look creamy. Later on it will look like thin, bluish nonfat cow's milk. The milk your baby gets during his first sucks is different from the "hind milk" that comes out last. Don't think it's not rich enough; your breastmilk is *perfect*.

## Nursing Positions

You'll soon find your favorite nursing positions.

- Make yourself cozy with pillows behind your back or under the baby. You might want to crank your hospital bed down a bit so you don't have to strain your muscles to hold either yourself or your infant. Keep two cloth diapers or towels nearby— one for your lap in case of diaper leaks, and another on your shoulder to catch any drips or spit-ups.

- Once you feel snug, nestle your baby's head in the crook of your arm and draw him next to your breast until you feel like you're belly-to-belly. Draw your nipple across his cheek. He will turn his head and root for it (a marvelous natural reflex). Now you can nestle him in closer.

- With your hand, guide your *entire* nipple into his mouth, keeping his nose free. Make sure he takes most of the dark area around the nipple, called the areola, as well. If he just nurses on the tip, you'll get sore nipples, and he won't get as much food for his work, since the areola empties its milk reserves into your nipple when his gums press down on them.

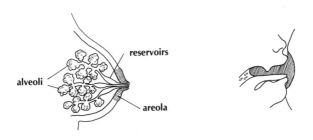

- Get a good firm grip on his leg or bottom so that he'll feel secure. Don't distract him—some babies are easily annoyed when they're trying to nurse and you're playing with their ears or toes.

- Let him nurse for about ten minutes on one side before interfering (checking his diaper or burping him). After you've changed sides, your baby can nurse as long as he'd like on the other breast.

**A newborn baby will empty a breast in about twenty minutes; older babies can finish much faster. But unless your breasts are sore, let him nurse longer to satisfy his sucking need.**

Your baby will soon set his own nursing schedule, so don't worry if you do nothing but rock, rest, and nurse the first few weeks. Liberal nursing guards you against infection, soreness (as long as the baby is positioned properly), and engorgement, and makes for a generous milk supply from the start.

When you want to take your baby off the breast, break the suction by gently inserting your finger between your breast and his lips. Some moms pull down on their baby's chin, but when I tried that mine just clamped down harder. At the next nursing, start him off on the side he last nursed on. Since he nursed longer on the last side, that breast will be fuller and will feel harder.

It can be hard to remember where you left off. Some moms keep a safety pin on their bra to mark the side most recently used. Or shift your wedding ring from left to right to remind yourself where to start. Since I tend to forget such things, I usually just feel which breast is more firm and start there. Your baby will then end up nursing longest on the breast less recently nursed.

Don't be alarmed if you feel cramping while you nurse. Your baby's early sucking releases a powerful maternal hormone (oxytocin) which causes the uterus to contract each time the baby nurses, bringing it back into its pre-pregnant shape. While helping to push out the placenta, oxytocin also reduces bleeding by closing off the blood vessels that were once attached to the placenta. So if you feel cramping, remember that you're actually healing yourself while feeding your baby.

## Nursing Lying Down

The lying-down position is a nursing favorite, perhaps because you can both fall asleep. It's an ideal way for a Caesarean mom to breastfeed her baby.

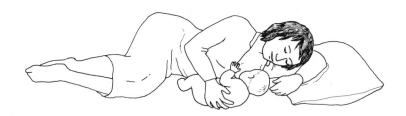

To breastfeed on the left side, lie down on your left side and put your left arm above the baby's head, or wherever it feels comfortable. Use your right arm to cuddle the baby in and bring his legs in close to you (this will help keep his nose clear).

Next, pull him yet closer until you feel his cheek next to your breast. He'll then root and suck. What a blissful way to nurse: he can fall asleep, and you won't have to worry about waking him up to lay him down somewhere.

Or you can simply lie down on your stomach with your arms crossed under your head or pillow. If you tilt up a bit on one side, your baby can nurse and you can sleep, too.

**Food for Thought.** Unfortunately for my husband and me, our oldest daughter was already eight months old before I read *The Family Bed* by Tine Thevinin. That book, plus the folks at La Leche League and advice from several pediatricians, inspired me to ignore the superstitions about nursing and sleeping with a baby. Some cultures still regard it as child abuse to separate a child from his mother and leave him in a room alone! In fact, it's only been in this century that we've turned to separate rooms and separate beds. Many moms keep the crib or bassinet next to their bed so they can easily bring their baby under the covers and nurse. Or they start their child out in his own bed and bring him in later in the night. Everybody gets more sleep, and parenting becomes simpler! Sleeping together is especially valuable to working parents who can gain that much more closeness with their baby. After all, who likes sleeping alone? As one mom says, "Just because it's dark outside doesn't mean that I should stop mothering my child!" The important thing is to love your baby and meet his needs, both day and night. ■

While you're still in the hospital, try to nurse both sitting up and lying down. You can also experiment with your own positions, such as the "football" hold in which your baby is cradled in one arm along the side of your body. A baby can nurse on your right breast if you cup him with your right arm along your right side. That hold comes in especially handy if your baby prefers to nurse on one side over the other, since you can simply change his position and use alternating breasts.

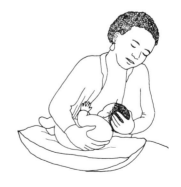

As far as nursing supplies go, you'll certainly travel lighter than a mom who has to carry bottles and formula. The only equipment needed are new bras for your bigger breast size, but don't buy those until after your baby is born and you can get an exact fit for your new figure. Also buy some cotton hankies or nursing pads to protect against leaking and a cotton towel or diaper in case of burping.

As discussed earlier, you don't need special clothes to nurse discreetly. Any two-piece outfit, with a top that can be pulled up, lets baby nurse as her body covers your partially bare midriff. Many mothers prefer just to push up their bra rather than fiddle with flaps on nursing bras. Regular clothes can also be easier than nursing garments with hidden openings and noisy Velcro closures.

---

## SOME COMMON NURSING PROBLEMS, AND HOW TO SOLVE THEM

| | |
|---|---|
| Sore nipples | Try shorter, more frequent nursings. |
| | Check your baby's nursing position; he should have your areola in his mouth. |
| | Dry your nipples before covering them. |
| | Expose your nipples to air, sunlamp (briefly). |
| | Rub in a bit of pure lanolin. |
| | Relax, then hand express to start your milk flow before your baby latches on. (See page 44.) |
| | Could be thrush, a common fungus infection. Consult your doctor. |
| Retracted nipples | True cases are very rare! |
| | Most inverted nipples stand out after being gently massaged and drawn out. |
| Sore breast (mom may have fever, chills, red streak on breast) | Check with your doctor: could be a plugged duct or an infection. |
| | Rest, and nurse your baby in bed with you. |
| | Apply heat, take a hot shower. |
| | Hand express some milk, then massage the sore area. |
| | Nurse more frequently on the sore side. |
| | Bra too tight? |
| Breasts too full (most often happens during first week of nursing) | Empty your breasts by nursing often. |
| | Express milk to relieve pressure. |
| | Take a hot shower. |
| | Use hot or cold compresses. |

| | |
|---|---|
| Not enough milk | Remember the law of supply and demand!<br>Increase nursing to increase supply; nurse at least every two hours.<br>Eat well, take prenatal vitamins, drink fluids.<br>Avoid supplementary bottles.<br>Relax, take a nap with baby.<br>Is baby happy? Thriving? Wetting six diapers a day? You're doing great!<br>If not, contact your physician. |
| Leaking/dripping milk | Use nursing pads/cotton hankies in your bra.<br>Apply pressure to your nipples to stop the flow.<br>Does your baby need to nurse? |
| Sick mother | Continue nursing, take your baby to bed.<br>Be sure your doctor prescribes medication suitable for nursing mothers, since substances do pass through your milk.<br>Drink plenty of liquids.<br>Don't worry about your baby getting sick. Breastmilk is protected by your immune system and your baby has an immune system of his own. |
| Sick baby | Continue nursing; it nourishes your baby and prevents dehydration.<br>Suction her nose if necessary to relieve stuffiness that prevents sucking.<br>Check with your pediatrician, especially before giving any medication, including aspirin.<br>A fussy baby could be reacting to something in *your* diet. |

Breastfeeding can be further delayed by hospital nurses who ask you to wash your hands and nipples (remember not to use soap or other drying agents which can cause your nipples to crack). I was once handed a large jar of cream and told to follow a five-step procedure before nursing my baby!

Such sterility is necessary in a hospital where there are unfamiliar germs and people. At home, your baby and you can both take it easier. Your regular daily shower will keep your breasts plenty clean.

If your baby chokes or gags while nursing, sit him up straight and he'll usually be fine. He might simply have let milk go down his breathing tube, or perhaps your milk came out so quickly he was too surprised to swallow!

You may have such a strong let-down reflex that your nipple squirts milk before he latches on. If you think your milk is coming out too fast and furious, express a little into a clean cloth diaper to reduce the flow.

## Burping

Some babies rarely need burping, while others need to be burped after each feeding. Often the simple act of lifting the baby to switch sides will bring up a bubble. If your baby falls asleep in your arm, don't wake her to burp! But if you think it's needed, put her head on your shoulder or lay her stomach down on your lap. She may like to be patted softly on her back. Or gently rock her in a sitting position on your lap, with your hands behind her back and neck.

If you have just nursed a "gulper" who swallowed a lot of air, be prepared for some milk to come up. Many parents wear a small towel or cotton diaper on their shoulder just in case.

## Vomiting

Your newborn might spit up after every nursing, especially when your milk supply has come in and is adjusting itself to her need. She simply eats too much and sends back what her stomach can't hold.

*Projectile* vomiting is when the milk is forcefully thrown out of the mouth rather than merely burped or spit up. If your baby repeatedly projectile vomits, call your doctor.

**Food for Thought.** Spitting up might be your baby's reaction to something in your diet. Our oldest daughter spit up and developed a diaper rash whenever I ate green peppers. Some pregnant or nursing moms who drink a lot of milk find out that their babies are allergic to dairy products, so they cut out milk for a few days to see if their infant feels better. If so, it's worth their effort to avoid milk and supplement their diets with extra calcium and protein, using lots of leafy greens, sesame and sunflower seeds, and soybean products such as soymilk and tofu. Other common allergens, such as wheat or corn, might also affect your baby. ■

If such dietary measures don't help, perhaps your baby is simply drinking more milk than her stomach can handle! Let her nurse longer on your empty breast, and hand express a bit of milk if you feel pressure.

## The Placid Baby

On the other hand, yours may be a placid baby who likes to sleep more than eat. Some babies thrive on less food than others; check with your doctor if you're concerned about your baby's weight. If your baby does need to nurse more often in order to gain weight, wake him up if he's sleeping longer than four hours at a stretch.

After all, newborns shouldn't be sleeping all night. Their tiny stomachs quickly digest breastmilk and need frequent refilling. Some babies who sleep through the night at a very early age may be satisfying their own needs by sucking their thumb or crying themselves back to sleep.

If you wake up and your breasts feel too full, bring your baby into bed to nurse. You'll feel relieved, and he won't wake up in pain from an empty stomach. And don't worry; both of you will soon have the instincts to know when you need each other to nurse. Once again, you're benefiting from the marvelous principle of supply and demand.

# Going Home: Your Family's New Needs

Of course, your hospital stay won't center entirely on breastfeeding. Ask a nurse to teach you how to diaper, bathe, and take over baby-caring duties so you'll be prepared at home.

Just before you check out, a nurse may hand you a goodie bag full of samples from baby companies. You'll probably get disposable diapers, nursing pads, coupons for baby photographers, and a ton of other advertisements.

**If you're breastfeeding, don't take home the sample cans of baby formula! Somebody might be tempted to use them. If you do take formula home, feed it to your cat.**

Finally, home sweet home. Your own familiar sheets, kitchen, noise, and mess. Dad or Grandma can hold the baby while you take a hot shower. Or you might prefer a sitz bath if you need to soothe hemorrhoids or an episiotomy.

Ignore the mess for a while. Get some outside cleaning assistance for at least a month if you can afford it. This kind of help, along with diaper service for those who don't use disposables, make a great gift from co-workers, groups of friends, and doting grandparents. Drop a few hints!

If people offer to bring meals or wash dishes, let them. This is no time to be a martyr; you need your rest to recover from labor and delivery, and to take on your new role as parent. Even if you usually have a hard time accepting love from others, show good manners by welcoming help and letting somebody feel useful.

In other words, don't ask others to hold your baby while you tackle the kitchen. You're probably feeling at least a few postpartum discomforts, which might continue for several months if you don't relax and adjust to your new life.

---

## Common Complaints After Birth:

**Constipation:** Don't strain, add fiber to your diet, take walks.

**Difficulty in emptying bladder:** Relax, drink more liquids

**Painful episiotomy stitches:** Hot bath, perhaps cream

**Cramps:** Your uterus is contracting; consult your doctor if the pain is extreme

**Engorged breasts:** More frequent nursing

**Sore nipples:** Check baby's nursing position, see advice on pages 32–35.

---

You'll need to wear a sterile sanitary napkin for your profuse, menstrual-like bleeding. That flow will be indicative of your recuperation: the initial bright red blood will turn brownish as your uterus heals itself. This is perhaps another one of the ways your body tells you to go easy. I once completely stopped bleeding two weeks after our son's birth, yet started again when he was five weeks old because I had resumed working with premature gusto.

This is the time you're most likely to overdo things. Your adrenaline and hormones are running sky-high, yet you're also dangerously close to exhaustion. One mom of six routinely keeps her robe on for a full six weeks after childbirth: "That way, I know not to run to the store, clean the house, or throw a party! And others know to let me rest, as well."

While most of us are out and about much before that, we still need to be careful. And don't be scared if you find yourself crying or overly emotional. Postpartum depression is very real as new moms experience hormonal swings.

**You're probably overdoing it if you**
- **resume a bright red flow**
- **have a sore breast, headache, or fever**
- **simply feel exhausted**

**Take your baby to bed!**

Things will be running at full tilt soon enough. It will take you two or three weeks before nursing is established. For now, get a good milk supply, and get your emotions under control before you even think about vacuuming.

Find your way back to your normal pattern as slowly and easily as you can. Many moms find that their milk won't flow if they're tense or stressed. Your let-down reflex depends on your peace of mind, and so does your baby. I've learned the hard way that there's nothing to make a baby cry like a hurried, tense parent.

As one new mother put it, "Here I was, trying to dazzle my in-laws with a spotless house, gourmet meals, and perfect grand-child. Yet neither my baby nor I could stop crying until I let everything slide, put my feet up, and nursed her. Once I listened to her, she showed me exactly what we both needed to do: cherish each other!"

# Spoiling Your Baby? Nonsense!

Babies cry for a lot of reasons; hunger, boredom, and pain, for example. You'll soon recognize the looks and special cry that go with each emotion. The important thing is to answer your baby as soon as she lets you know that something's wrong.

Go to her whenever she cries so that she'll know she can depend on you to nurse or hold her. And ignore anybody who implies that your precious newborn is manipulating you into spoiling her forever. Isn't it a little early to suspect that your new child is trying to mislead you?

A crying baby is usually asking for something that's easily given. Maybe she needs burping or more time at the breast, or perhaps she's reacting to something in your diet or those new infant vitamins. If nursing isn't the answer, put her in a frontpack and she'll probably quiet down as she senses your warmth and movement.

Such quiet solutions can be the key to relaxed, successful nursing, as well as your baby's feeling of self-worth. As your child grows, she will continually ask for your reassuring attention. Your ready and loving responses to her help shape her own feelings of security and confidence.

"The very fact that so many babies are now carried about is reflected in new child development trends of brightness and sharpness," says Marian Thompson, co-founder of La Leche League. "When he's at shoulder level, his brain will be stimulated by the colors, sounds, and people you're seeing. And you'll be much more aware of his needs, as well."

In short: *hold your baby!* And take her with you wherever you go. She'll soon be squirming to get out of your arms, so enjoy what cuddling you can. Your warm embrace, along with clean diapers and your nursing, is about all that she needs right now for true happiness! Not much to ask, is it?

# Mom's Diet: As Important As Ever

It's true: your diet needs to be as superior as when you were pregnant. As a nursing mother, you need to drink at least a quart more fluid and eat about one-fourth more solid food than you did before you were pregnant, which amounts to about 1,000 extra calories per day.

Not only do you need extra calories while nursing, you need energy-packed food to regain your strength. Yet you also need to rely on your slow-cooker and simple dishes so that you'll have the most time possible to enjoy your baby.

Continue your prenatal vitamins and food to grow on. Some handy fortifiers are wheat germ and brewer's yeast for B complex vitamins and E, molasses for iron and B vitamins, and yogurt for B vitamins and vitamin K.

You may also need extra fiber in your diet, especially if you've had an episiotomy and are having trouble with constipation. Try eating an apple before bedtime, and enjoy a bran muffin or whole grain cereal with dried fruit for breakfast.

Perhaps most important is your need for fluids. You need about three quarts of fluid each day to make quality breastmilk. Don't drink so much that you feel uncomfortable, but you probably need more fluids than before you were pregnant. Grab a tall glass of water and a high-protein snack every time you sit down to nurse. And some extra nibbling on whole foods can do wonders for your energy and milk supply.

**Now's the time to encourage the rest of your family to enjoy whole foods, if you haven't already. You'll all have more energy if you eat right. Before you know it, six months will fly by and your baby will be ready for solid food from your table.**

Just as substances passed through your placenta to your baby, they also pass through your breastmilk. Caffeine, alcohol, medications, and smoking are dangerous for your newborn. According to Paul Fleiss, M.D., "In breastmilk of smoking mothers, we can find levels of the cancer-causing chemical, benzopyrene. And alcohol can be just as destructive to your baby's brain cells as it is to yours."

New moms were once advised to relax with a glass of beer or wine. Now we know that we should actually think twice about alcohol's long-term effects.

# Nursing Under Special Circumstances

Whether you're going back to work or nursing a premature baby, breastfeeding can present special challenges. Hospitalization or daycare may require a mom to pump her breasts, both for milk storage and for keeping up her supply.

Hand expression is generally much easier than using mechanical pumps. One manual technique (Marmet) includes massage and stimulation to assist your let-down reflex, which isn't as strong as when a baby directly nurses.

First, picture how your milk is produced. After its creation in cells called alveoli, milk constantly comes through your breast ducts into reservoirs just under your darker-skinned areola. More milk is sent into the duct system during the let-down reflex, when milk-producing cells are stimulated.

To further drain your milk reservoirs, you need to stimulate the flow of milk by helping your let-down reflex. You may only want to express to relieve pressure in too-full breasts. I found the Marmet technique especially helpful to drain an occasional plugged duct or breast infection. (This is also much gentler than one of those horn-shaped manual pumps.)

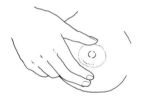

## How to Hand-Express Your Milk or Colostrum: The Marmet Technique

1. Put your thumb above the nipple and your first two fingers below and about one inch behind the nipple.
2. Without spreading your fingers, push straight in toward your chest.
3. Roll your thumb and fingers forward. Pretend you're making fingerprints.
4. The entire procedure should be repeated according to this pattern: position, push, roll. Use both hands on each breast, and change positions to drain other milk reservoirs.

With this technique, you'll avoid the bruising, skin burns, and tissue damage of other hand-expression methods. The key is to avoid the squeezing, hand sliding, and pulling out on the nipple and breast that can come from over-eager expressing.

Your breasts will react just as if your baby were nursing; the more your reservoirs are drained, the more milk will be produced to refill them. Once you've expressed milk for about five minutes, your reservoirs will usually be drained.

If you want more milk, you'll need to stimulate the flow by assisting your let-down reflex. This procedure is much like routine breast exams:

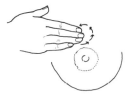

# How to Stimulate
# Your Let-Down Reflex

1.  Massage the milk cells and ducts by moving your fingers in a circular motion in one spot. After a few seconds, move to another spot until you've massaged the entire area.
2.  Relax your reflex by stroking the entire breast with light motions from the chest wall to the nipple.
3.  Lean your breasts forward and shake them. Gravity can help your milk travel into your ducts.

The above procedure takes twenty to thirty minutes. You might try it in a hot shower your first few times, until you get a feel for the technique and how your milk comes out. Don't worry if no milk comes out during your first attempts.

Here is a suggested timing for breasts with apparently little or no milk: express each breast for five minutes or until the flow of milk (if there is any) slows down. Then massage, stroke, and shake each breast at the same time. Re-express each breast for three to five minutes, and repeat the massage, stroke, shake let-down. Finally, express each breast for another two or three minutes.

If you're planning to leave your baby and you need to express enough milk for one feeding, start to express your milk at least twenty-four hours before going out. Express only after each nursing, and store the milk in a sterilized bottle in the refrigerator.

I've seen this marvelous method work for many moms who need to bottle their breast milk. It's even helped adoptive moms *who've never breastfed before* make enough milk to at least partially nurse their babies!

If you have no luck with hand expressing, there are modern electric pumps and a device called "Lact-Aid" to help you. Ask your hospital nurse or pediatrician about local sources for this equipment.

## Storing Your Milk

Your doctor or hospital staff can show you methods for storing your expressed milk. Cleanliness is your major concern, so be careful not to handle the inside or top of any container.

In one case, the mom of a preemie was given bottles of sterile water which she emptied. Then she filled each bottle with her milk, either by expressing it directly or first expressing it into a sterile specimen cup.

Many mothers immediately label the bottle with their baby's name and date of expression. Keep it in the refrigerator if you're going to use it within the next day or two. Otherwise, it must be quickly frozen. Frozen milk keeps for at least two weeks in a refrigerator ice-cube compartment. But why worry? Use your expressed milk as soon as possible.

To thaw frozen breastmilk, put the bottle under cold running water, then gradually warm it until it liquifies. You can heat it in a pan of water on your stove top. It should be comfortably warm when you test a drop on your wrist. *Don't let it thaw by standing at room temperature.*

## Breastfeeding After A Caesarean Section

If yours is a planned birth, find out everything you can before the big event. Caesarean sections are increasingly common, and most hospitals are now encouraging the father to be present. Even if *you* can't hold your baby right after delivery, Dad can!

You can still nurse just as successfully as other mothers. Let your doctor and nurses know that you're anxious to start breastfeeding as soon as possible. A catheter and I.V. won't hamper your success: simply put your baby to breast and keep her there.

Your feeding positions may turn out to be remarkably simple since you don't have to sit up either to breastfeed or to burp. Your baby and you, aided with a few pillows, can find the way that suits you best.

Many moms prefer their bed to be nearly flat, with the bed rails up to help them roll over. To change nursing sides, just roll the baby over your chest.

Since you'll be in the hospital longer than most moms, request rooming-in, or at least an "on-demand" feeding arrangement. If you need pain medication, ask your doctor for one that won't affect your baby. And try to get up and around as soon as you can, breathing deeply. Life may seem a bit rocky during the second and third day after birth, but most moms perk up soon after that.

**If you're a diabetic mother, you are a prime candidate for a C-section, and you need to prepare yourself beforehand. Breastfeeding is especially advantageous to a diabetic mother, says Dr. Ruth A. Lawrence. Not only can lactation improve your health, but nursing your child immediately after birth may also prevent infant hypoglycemia. Follow the directions of your doctor, who can best advise you about your diet and other special concerns.**

Once home, remember that you need outside help and extra support more than ever. If money is a problem, remind yourself about how much you're saving by not buying bottles and formula. Somebody you feel comfortable with, such as Dad, Grandma, or a hired housekeeper, should always be with you to tend to the household.

Naps, fluids, and bed rest will greatly hasten your recovery. Follow your doctor's orders to recover from surgery, and your womanly instincts to breastfeed your baby. Although you may need to avoid painful cuddling, your nursing can be a gentle, loving joy for the whole family!

## Breastfeeding the Hospitalized Baby

Countless moms have met the challenges of nursing a hospitalized baby, even after months of I.V.s, oxygen, and surgery. While high-tech medical equipment may be keeping your child alive, it's your loving presence that can make a difference in his desire to live! Many doctors will encourage you to stay with your hospitalized baby, perhaps in the same room with her.

As soon as possible, breastfeed your baby with as much skin-to-skin contact as you can. Even without milk, nursing can be a precious time for the two of you. When your baby is ready to graduate from tube-feeding, tell your doctor that you prefer to eliminate bottles entirely by moving straight to breastfeeding.

If your baby can't suck, hand express or pump your breasts to build up your milk supply. Start as soon as you can after birth, and express every two hours. If your baby can't have your milk yet, donate it to other mothers or a hospital milk bank so that another child can get off to a better start.

Keep up your hopes and humor! Remember that even a "normal" nursing couple takes at least a month to establish a good routine. The more your baby sucks, the more milk you will have. And don't forget your vitamins and food to grow on to keep up your energy and great breastmilk.

When you finally wean from bottle to breast, thanks to your diligent pumping, your baby will be used to the taste of your milk. But he'll probably have some nipple confusion before he knows the milk is now coming out of you rather than a bottle.

Give a bottle only after nursing, and be sure to nurse as long as possible at each breast. You might want to feed your baby every two hours for the first few days at home, and over the course of a week shift to bottle-free, demand breastfeeding.

True, it's more work. But so worth it! Even if you don't nurse your hospitalized baby, your nearness and touch is the best mothering medicine he can get. Every child is born with his own strengths and weaknesses, and you can help give him the best possible start.

## Nursing and Going Back to Work

Not long ago, mothers stayed home with their children for the first three years. Taking a child outside the home for daycare was almost unknown, and sometimes thought to cause later neuroses.

Today, longer maternity leaves and nursing, working moms are much more common. Most women now breastfeed for at least six months instead of using the once-popular "dry-up" pills. Even if your employer only offers a six-week maternity leave, you can nurse at least that long, and even much longer!

Remind yourself of the reasons why breastfeeding is superior to formula. It certainly won't bog down your busy schedule, since you have to feed your baby anyway. Most nursing moms find their after-work nursing a special time to relax, forget outside pressures, and enjoy their baby.

Once you return to work, you can still keep up your regular nighttime, early morning, and evening feedings. Your only problem, in fact, is maintaining daytime nursings. Simply ask your babysitter to use bottles of your expressed milk.

> **Start to pump or express and store milk a week or so before you go back to work. By then you'll have a good idea of how many bottles you'll need, as well as how much milk to pump.**

One friend carried a sterile bottle to work with her each day. During breaks, she would go into the restroom and express milk into the bottle, then store it in the office refrigerator. That bottle was then fed to her child the next day, and often by Mom during a lunch break.

If your office situation makes pumping impossible, perhaps your babysitter can bring your child to you for some nursings. The location of your daycare center can be a major factor in its selection: it's sure nice to have your child close enough to visit.

Whether you breastfeed or not, your baby needs you. You're the only person who knows intuitively what he needs. Even though there may not always be perfect answers or situations, we can do our best by giving our babies our most loving care.

# Tips For Formula-Feeding

Even though breast is best, it's not for everybody. There may be many reasons to turn to bottle-feeding, such as severe illness, prolonged separation from your baby, or problems arising after the birth. Some women simply find the whole idea of nursing unpleasant. Yet that doesn't necessarily make them less loving, nurturing mothers!

Whether your baby is fed by breast or bottle, it's important for his feeding time to be warm and intimate. Give him the reassuring warmth of your body and the smooth touch of your skin. Experts think such caressing gives a baby the feel of the uterus lining, as well as his mother's familiar heartbeat, voice, and movement.

Though you may at times feel rushed and harried, don't get in the habit of propping his bottle. He not only will miss your closeness and security, but more important, he might spit up or choke while feeding. You must be there to be sure he doesn't aspirate the formula into his lungs. Even a six-month-old who can hold his own bottle should be supervised.

## Finding the Best Formula

Ask your doctor about which formula to use for your infant. Most commercial formulas are as similar as possible in composition to breast milk, although you may go through a period of trial and error in finding a suitable brand if your child is allergic to cow's milk or other common formula ingredients.

**No matter which formula you choose, be sure it is the one best suited for your baby. Common symptoms of allergy or milk intolerance include stomach cramps, rash, or red, sore bottom. In such cases, contact your doctor. Tests will reveal if your baby needs a special non-cow's-milk formula with a soybean, meat protein, or alternative base. You should also check with your doctor before switching brands of formula.**

Several companies offer natural products for the varying needs of pregnant and nursing women, newborns, infants, weaning babies, and toddlers. Ask your doctor if she is familiar with some of the newest natural prepared formulas (such as those from Sunshine and Rainbow) which contain barley to aid in whole milk digestion as well as full complements of vitamins, minerals, and protein. (See listings in Recommended Readings and Resources.)

For whatever reason you don't nurse your baby, you can still give him as wholesome and superior a formula as possible.

# Preparing the Bottle

Cleanliness is a key element in preparing a bottle for your baby, so be sure to follow the formula manufacturer's directions for mixing and storage. It is crucial that all equipment and formula be properly sterilized and handled, *so ask your doctor or nurse to tell you the best way to do this.* Nowadays, most doctors recommend using dishwashers or hot soapy water to clean bottles.

Some pediatricians, including Dr. Graydon Funke, tell their patients not to bother with sterilization if they're using powdered formula and tap or bottled water to make a bottle for immediate feeding. "It's only when you're mixing up several bottles at a time, or the bottle will stand for over twenty minutes, that you need to worry about bacteria with powdered formula," Funke says.

Many parents use the "aseptic" method when they need to sterilize bottles. All the equipment (bottle, cap, nipple, spoon) is sterilized before the formula is mixed. You can boil them for half an hour in a covered saucepan, or use a sterilizer unit. Another option is to use a liquid or tablet to sterilize enough water to cover all the equipment in a special container. The formula is then mixed in the bottles with boiled, cooled water.

With the "terminal" method, formula is first mixed in the bottle with cold tap water. A clean nipple is placed upside-down in the bottle neck, which is then loosely capped to allow steam to pass through. Bottles are then placed (right side up) in about four inches of water in a saucepan or sterilizer. The unit is covered, water boils for about half an hour, and the bottles are allowed to cool (still covered) for several hours.

Many formulas may be prepared in sufficient quantity to fill enough bottles for an entire day. Any filled bottles not needed immediately must be refrigerated and not stored for more than twenty-four hours. Leftover formula should not be reheated.

In addition to an ample supply of formula, you will also need about six bottles of various sizes made from heat-resistant plastic or glass. For example, you can use small bottles for water, unsweetened fruit juice, or breastmilk. Larger bottles come with either a wide neck (easier to clean with a bottle brush) or small neck (baby may swallow less air with her milk). If you decide to use plastic bags to hold the formula, remember that the disposable sacs fit into straight-sided bottles.

You will find it much easier if all your bottles, formula, and other baby-feeding equipment are stored in one place in your kitchen, preferably near the sink, stove, and flat working surface.

---

# Equipment for Your Bottle Feeding Center

- Six or more bottles, nipples, and caps
- Pint jar with cover to hold nipples
- Long metal spoon to mix formula
- Measuring cup
- Can opener
- Measuring cup or pitcher
- Scoop if using dry formula
- Two or more bottle brushes
- Bottle warmer or saucepan to hold warm water
- Bottle sterilizing unit or deep kettle
- Sterilizing tablets

---

Of course, be sure to follow the precise manufacturer's instructions in preparing any formula. Mixing too little formula with water may malnourish your child, while too much formula in the water causes an over-concentration that can be harmful. Adding extra sweetening can cause stomach upsets and excess weight gain, unless you are making your own formula under the guidance of your pediatrician.

## How to Give a Bottle

Wash your hands first thing, even before taking the bottle from the refrigerator. Your baby may not even want the milk warmed, or you can quickly heat it by placing the bottle in a saucepan of water over heat, or in a pitcher of hot water. Before giving the bottle to baby, sprinkle a few drops of formula on your wrist to be sure it is not too hot. The liquid should feel about the same temperature as your skin.

When bubbles rise in the formula as baby sucks, you know he is getting milk for his efforts. If he quickly loses interest or becomes fussy, perhaps the milk is flowing out too slowly. Check to be sure that the bottle cap is not secured too tightly, and that the rubber nipple is firm.

Or perhaps the nipple hole is too small. You can enlarge it with a hot needle that you've held over a flame and then quickly inserted. A new nipple may need several insertions. Be sure to sterilize it before using.

To test the size of the nipple hole, hold the bottle upside down and let the milk drip on your wrist. It should come out in large, single drops rather than in a constant stream. If the milk streams out, the nipple hole is too large and the nipple should be discarded. Babies who try to drink too much milk often swallow a lot of air and are soon fussy, choking, or spitting up.

To feed your baby, simply hold him close and cuddle him as if you were breastfeeding. While he sucks, hold the bottle at whatever angle allows the milk to fill the nipple and neck of the bottle. This will help your baby swallow more milk and less air, which means no painful burping. (See page 38 for ways to burp your baby.)

If your baby enjoys a nighttime bottle, give him one of water rather than formula or juice. You will be preventing future tooth decay, since the salivary process of a sleeping child slows down and does not wash away the sweet liquid which can attack his teeth.

# Common Myths About Babies, Bottles, and Breastmilk

**Myth.** "Your baby will choke if allowed to nurse after birth. Better to give him a sip of water."

**Your Answer.** "Any mucus in a baby's throat is likely to be coughed or sneezed up. In fact, colostrum will help wash it down."

**Myth.** "Your baby should drink from a bottle so you can measure how much she's eating and if it's enough. How else can you be sure you have enough milk?"

**Your Answer.** "My doctor can weigh her and measure her progress. She's happy, thriving, and has about six wet diapers a day. Since she nurses on demand, I'm confident she's getting all she needs. Besides, a newborn doesn't regain her birth weight for two or three weeks."

**Myth.** "Your baby needs sugar water or formula from a bottle."

**Your Answer.** "Breastmilk and colostrum have *all* the natural nutrients my baby needs, and are much easier for her to digest!"

**Myth.** "You should get your baby used to a bottle so you can leave her when you want to go out."

**Your Answer.** (Who's the parent here, anyway? You've worked too hard for this baby to leave her while she still needs you so much!) "Nursing is the easiest, most convenient, and healthiest way to feed our baby. And she's so easy to satisfy that she can go anywhere with us!"

## For Friendly Support

Parenting is natural, but that doesn't mean you can do it all by instinct. Perhaps you can start a support group with the women you met in your childbirth preparation class. Even if you're not nursing, you can learn more about mothering at La Leche League meetings.

LLL is an international, non-profit, non-sectarian organization. Local groups usually meet monthly to cover such topics as advantages and techniques of breastfeeding, identifying and overcoming difficulties, and nursing beyond infancy. A host of other interests are also discussed, ranging from first foods to discipline.

If you need some advice or words of encouragement, call one of LLL's volunteer leaders. These mothers are trained, accredited women who have nursed their own babies and enjoy helping others give their babies the best start in life. Some common advice: "Stick with it! You can do it! Relax, cheer up, and call if you need me!"

For me, LLL has been an invaluable support group and resource, and a great way to meet other families! Whether you need tips on returning to work or you have a husband who feels left out, you'll find a group of caring people who make parenting a lot easier.

Check in the white pages of your telephone directory for the nearest chapter, or write to the national office: La Leche League International, Inc., 9616 Minneapolis Ave., Franklin Park, Illinois 60131.

# Vitamins and Fluoride: When to Start?

The issue of when to start (or stop) vitamins with children is hopelessly tangled. You can call twenty doctors and get twenty different answers. Some doctors start babies at two weeks, while others wait until six months.

On one hand, the Committee on Nutrition of the American Academy of Pediatrics advises *against* supplements past infancy for healthy children who eat normal diets. The committee believes that if you're well-nourished and nursing your baby, or using an approved formula with supplements already in it, your baby is getting all the nutrients he needs. Even extra water is deemed unnecessary.

"We should get our vitamins naturally from the foods we eat," says Dr. Bart Asner, a pediatrician and spokesperson for the American Academy of Pediatrics. He goes on to say that nursing moms pass along their vitamin supplements through breastmilk. In fact, many of the obscure ingredients on the label of a formula can are added vitamins.

Some doctors recommend a fluoride drop supplement with vitamins A, C, and D for babies more than six months old. Such vitamins (but not fluoride) are often stopped after a child's first birthday, unless sickness or a medication causes a deficiency. Other doctors advise people of all ages to take vitamin supplements.

If your pediatrician suggests a liquid vitamin for your newborn, ask about using a natural alternative as opposed to the commercial brands. Dr. Lendon Smith believes that "it is probably better to use cod-liver oil as the infant's source of vitamin A (5000 to 10,000 units per day) and D (500 to 1000 units per day) than the vitamins in a base with sugar, color, and flavorings."

**In most cases, giving a healthy, breastfed baby vitamins or minerals is unnecessary if his mother is well-nourished. In fact, liquid supplements are often routinely prescribed simply so parents will remember to give their baby fluoride! Talk with your doctor to determine what's best before starting any vitamin program.**

**Food for Thought.** Nursing moms, remember to take *your* vitamins! And check with your doctor to be sure they are the right ones in the correct dosages, for your sake as well as for your baby's health and intelligence. The brain cells of your newborn will continue to multiply until he's about six months old. He depends entirely on your nutrition during that time. ■


## Fluoride: the Tooth Toughener

There's no doubt about it; nearly everybody praises fluoride. Pediatric dentists, now armed with new rinses, mouthwashes, and fluoridated tap water, are even predicting that cavities will be gone within ten years.

Your child's need for fluoride increases as he gets older. Some dentists advise tablets for six-week-old babies who are forming their permanent teeth. Your pediatrician might want to give your breastfed infant extra fluoride, or might recommend that you drink fluoridated water to toughen his unerupted teeth.

But, "it's difficult to predict how much fluoride each child gets, especially as they get older," says Dr. Denis Weintraub, pediatric dentist. "A child drinking bottled water, for example, won't be getting the same amount as one drinking lots of fluoridated tap water."

Your pediatrician can guide you in prescribing how much fluoride your family needs. Call your local water company to see how much fluoride, if any, is added to your water. You might need more than you're getting, especially if you use a reverse osmosis water filter (which filters out both salt and fluoride from your water). Fluoride also comes in most toothpastes, dental treatments, and natural sources such as shellfish.

Dr. Asner says that, "as a general rule, extra fluoride is needed for infants who are either breastfed or who take ready-to-feed formula. But if you're mixing concentrated formula with fluoridated tap water, you're probably getting enough."

Many doctors prescribe a daily .25 mg. dosage of fluoride during a child's first year. Ask your pediatrician about other dosages, and whether the fluoride should be given along with some form of magnesium or calcium.

# Confidential to Dad
# (Mom Should Read, Too!)

This is probably the most topsy-turvy time of your life; your "baby blues" are just as real as the hormonal craziness of your mate. (In fact, her postpartum depression has been clinically compared to combat fatigue.) You may feel demoted to chief bottlewasher and gofer as your wife and baby recover from birth. But believe me, whatever you give out will come back to you a hundred times over!

For example, it may be up to you to limit visitors if she's showing signs of weariness or if she just needs to relax. She'll need your support and protection when Aunt Molly asks, "Why are you nursing? Your husband wasn't nursed, and he turned out great!"

In the face of such real (and imagined) pressures, be prepared for emotional outbursts, and step in on her behalf. She's extremely sensitive to what you think, and she needs to sense your willingness to support her. Just knowing that you're pleased with and proud of her can help her cope with new demands and erratic schedules.

- Help her to regain her strength.
- Gently discourage her from overdoing during that crucial first month.
- Encourage frequent nursing, since it's a great excuse for her to relax and put her feet up.
- Give her a special back massage, or surprise her with a new book to read.

My husband once took our older children on a shopping spree. They came back with an organized diaper bag complete with baby wipes, changing pad, and small trash bags.

You'll both need to wait until the doctor gives his O.K. for sexual intercourse. Even then, it will be a lot different than it was in pre-baby days; a mom who's just healed from an episiotomy has been sewn back into a virginal tightness! And, although breastfeeding may cause temporary baby spacing, it's not a reliable means of birth control. Slowly and gently is the key.

You can help your child get the best possible breastmilk. Quietly hand your wife a glass of water and a nutritious snack, or refill her water pitcher when you sense she needs more liquids.

Remember to slip a casserole into the oven at four o'clock so she can concentrate on loving your baby.

Peace of mind is the best gift you can give her. If she is discouraged about nursing, call your local La Leche League chapter (it's listed in the phone book) and hand her the phone for some free mother-to-mother advice. You'll hear some comforting words for yourself, as well.

Never underestimate your new role as a father! Your masculine voice can do wonders at soothing the "five-o'clock fussies," and your strong, capable hands are true blessings during burpings, baths, and diaper changes. Lay down next to your child and watch him snuggle next to you. The more involved the dad, the better the kid!

This is an extraordinary chance for you to give of yourself and literally make a world of difference. So even if nobody else does, pat yourself on your back. You're needed now more than ever before!

---

# FUN IN THE KITCHEN

*Dishes that give you energy and time to enjoy your baby, plus some nice ideas for company.*

Breadcrust Zucchini Quiche

Crabby Mousse

Cranberry Apple Glog

Slow-Cooker Beans

Easiest Ever Granola

Honey Carob Chip Ice Cream

Iced Herbal Sun Tea

Peanut Butter Cookies for a Crowd

Pumpkin Butter

Tangy Lemon Fish

Wallace's Breakfast Drink

Your Own Peanut Butter Cups

---

# 3 FEEDING YOUR SOCIABLE SIX-MONTH-OLD

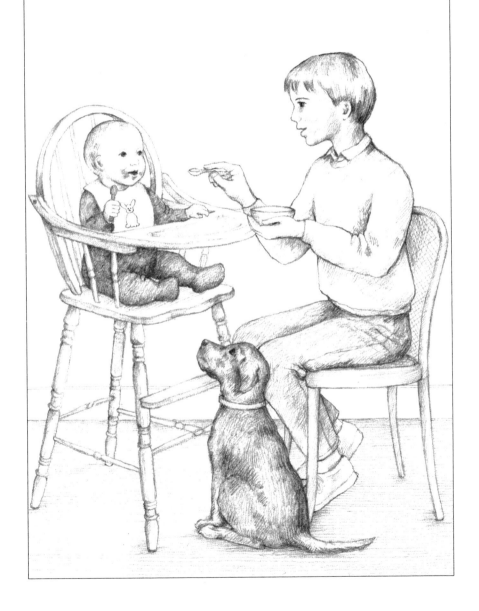

- sit up without support, crawl, and begin to walk
- reach for objects, then hold, examine, and throw them
- babble to you and understand many things you say
- cut between two to six teeth
- become easily distracted during nursings
- delight in new foods and his new-found coordination as he attempts to feed himself

**S**UCH CHANGE in six months! Your newborn is now an active member of the family, laughing at jokes, trying to sit up by herself, and grabbing morsels off your dinner plates. You may have friends who are asking, "What? You haven't given your baby solid food yet? Can't you tell she's *hungry?*"

But remind yourself that you're still offering the most perfect food you can give your baby for at least the first year. By holding off on solids, you're giving her immature digestive system time to grow ready for other foods.

Your baby is probably ready for solids if:

- She is about six months old or more
- She isn't satisfied with extra feedings
- She's chewing toys for hunger rather than for relief of her sore, teething gums
- She's eyeing your lunch!

According to the American Academy of Pediatrics, six months can be a magic age for a baby's nutritional needs. First, the iron supply that you gave your child before her birth is nearly gone, so she may need extra nutrients. Second, after a half-year of being strengthened with breastmilk, her digestive system is mature enough to start drawing nutrients from other foods.

"Actually, the only logical reason for starting solids earlier than six months is to keep babies from getting milk anemia, which comes only from cow's milk," says Dr. Lendon Smith. "Wait till your baby starts grabbing food off your plate or gets teeth. By delaying solids, you'll reduce the chance of allergy which many babies can never outgrow!"

Of course, all babies don't sit up and ask for food on their six-month birthday. Some wiry, active babies may need something a month earlier, while others will refuse to swallow anything until they walk.

Our oldest daughter could hardly wait to slurp some squash at five months old, yet her younger sister wanted simply to gnaw on a carrot stick until she was eight months along, when she *literally* pounced on a roast chicken.

**Food for Thought.** You may be getting your first glimpses of competition between parents, especially between those of first born children. In their craving to have a perfect child, some parents race to have their child be the *first* to sleep through the night, start solid foods, or take a first step. In five years, those same kids may be pushed to be the top reader, best dresser, best *everything*. Ignore such pressure by simply allowing your baby to be a baby. Just as you respect her needs about nursing, you can lovingly teach her how to enjoy food to grow on at her own pace. ■

# First Steps Toward Solids

Even if you are reasonably sure that your baby is ready to start solid foods, keep breastmilk or formula as the priority food for the first year. You'll keep up your milk supply if you nurse *before* mealtimes.

Some parents feed their baby during the more peaceful times of the day, such as mid-afternoon when they don't have to worry about serving everybody at once. As one mom puts it, "When I first fed Justin solids, I wanted to give him my full attention rather than try to feed his father, sister, and myself at the same time."

On the other hand, I found it easier to eat all together, since a sociable six-month-old wants to be included with everybody else. Once a baby is ready for solids, he knows that a toy on his highchair tray just doesn't cut it. He wants to join in the fun!

# Tools of the Trade

Now's the time to get a sturdy **highchair** or **clamp-on seat** that allows baby to sit at the table with the rest of the family. Not all equipment is well-designed, so look for the safest when shopping for any baby accessory, including strollers and carriers.

When choosing a highchair, look for:
- a chair with a wide base that keeps it stable
- a safety belt that attaches to the frame rather than the tray
- a tray that latches securely on both sides
- mechanisms and parts that are free of sharp points and edges

Don't think you have to buy an expensive wooden model with ten adjustments and hand-painted teddy bears; it will soon be buried beneath a layer of mashed carrots and grape juice stains. Just as your baby explores your house, he will also delight in seeing how well peas squish and bananas smear.

Use a **non-breakable bowl** and buy a **small, non-breakable plastic spoon** that he can hold himself. (Eventually, he'll grab it out of your hand and make spectacular messes while trying to feed himself.) Some baby spoons are shaped like tiny bowls at one end, while others have a curved handle that fits well into a tiny palm.

Next, **prepare your surroundings** for disaster. If you're the carefree sort and the highchair is on a washable surface, you can simply put a bib on your baby and let 'er rip. Or perhaps you'll rest easier if the chair is over an old shower curtain or sheet. If the weather is warm and the food unusually messy (bananas, for instance), you can simply strip baby down to his diaper and plan on a bath after dinner.

Since first foods are often mashed and spoonfed, you may want to buy an inexpensive **baby food grinder**. Choose one that's small and easy to clean; you can tuck it in a diaper bag along with a bib, spoon, and bowl. Another optional luxury is a **blender** for whirling baby foods and preparing frothy drinks.

When I was feeding our first baby, I swore by my baby food grinder. Yet with subsequent children, and a lack of time to leisurely plan infants' meals, I simply used a fork to mash foods. It was easier, quicker, and more efficient, especially since babies love to pick up peas and other finger foods. Mashed food also introduces children to different textures and the joys of chewing or gumming from the start.

As your baby becomes used to eating, you can place her food right on her plate. But food should never be spooned directly from a baby food jar into your child's mouth. The saliva from a spoon dipped back into a jar can spread bacteria throughout the food. Transfer the amount of food you need into a bowl and throw away any leftovers.

## Your Home-Cooked Fare Is Great!

With the start of solids, your baby will be eating foods that aren't as easy to digest as breastmilk. Add foods, therefore, that are as nutritiously pure and close to breastmilk as possible.

Start your baby on your everyday, home-cooked whole foods. Not only will you spare yourself the tremendous expense of canned baby foods, but you'll also get him used to the taste of nutritious fare.

True, the baby foods companies have cut down on salt, modified food starch, and sugar in their products, but it's so easy to gain complete control over the quality of your baby's food by making it yourself. Plus, as he develops more teeth and enjoys a greater selection of solids, he'll make an easy jump to enjoying whatever you're eating. No factory can produce food to equal your home cooking.

> **Plan ahead for those times when your family is dining on curry or other "grown-up" food. Next time you steam a vegetable or fix a stew, freeze a little extra in an ice cube tray and cover it with foil. You'll have a pint-sized meal all ready to thaw and serve!**

There's a good chance that your six-month-old may be ready to plunge right into finger-feeding. Simply put bits of food on the highchair tray or on an unbreakable plate; he'll be thrilled to develop his "pincer" ability of the thumb and index finger. Some babies so love to feed themselves that they won't accept any food from you until they can handle the spoon themselves.

## First Experiences With Food

If your baby seems too young for anything but spoonfeeding, try holding him on your lap and gently letting a tiny bit of food slip from a spoon into his mouth. He'll be amazed and confused by the sensations. Not only will he feel a hard, cold spoon in his mouth, but a new, mushy taste as well.

He's also developing a whole new set of muscles that he hasn't used in breastfeeding. A nursing infant uses his tongue to press the breast's nipple against the top of his mouth. This sucking reflex, which has served him so well in the past, will actually push out solid food! He'll try to nurse a spoon by clamping on it; no wonder his eyes widen with surprise!

---

### The Correct Amount

Offer only a teaspoon of a single food once or twice a day for three or four days before you move on to another item. Watch for signs of allergy:

- Red diaper area
- Runny nose
- Wheezing

---

You'll find that only the most passive babies will let themselves be overfed. After all, a baby doesn't feel morally obligated to finish his vegetable before dessert, or clean up his plate before leaving the table. (Older kids shouldn't be asked to eat more than they desire, either.)

A baby or toddler is in full rein of his own instincts. If you doubt this, just try to coax one more bite of applesauce into a baby that's had enough. He'll either angrily turn his head away or spit the food all over you! Pushing for "just one more bite" is a way to start overeating habits.

"Don't worry," he's telling you. " I've had my share. Just believe me." And so we should.

# Foods to Begin With

Your child's first solids must be the most pure, nutritious foods you can prepare. Not only are you giving your baby the taste of food to grow on, but you're also attempting to give him the vitamins, natural fats, and other properties of breastmilk.

Some doctors still recommend starting with a bland rice cereal, moistened with water or breastmilk. If yours does, choose a one-grain cereal rather than a multi-grain so you can pinpoint any problems. Yet the "start with cereal" theory could be a hangover from the old wives' tale about feeding your baby cereal that will "stick to his ribs and make him sleep through the night."

**Most of that cereal comes right out the other end. And, believe me, starting solids won't magically transform a baby into a twelve-hour sleeper. Your baby still needs to nurse on demand, and should continue to do so.**

---

## Perfect First Foods

- Steamed squash or other yellow vegetable
- In-season steamed veggies, such as squash or other yellow vegetable (but nothing astringent, such as rhubarb or beet greens)
- Mashed banana, finely grated raw apple
- Other in-season fruits, except for berries
- Whole grain toast crusts or unsweetened cereal
- Combinations of foods, such as applesauce/squash
- Lean, well-cooked meat, finely chopped, or hand your baby a chicken bone to gnaw on, minus the cartilage and skin

---

Bright colors, such as bits of young carrots and ripe cantaloupe seem to have a compelling attraction for little appetites. Our son loves to feed himself anything he sees his sisters eat, and often plays with an entire potato throughout dinner.

Several parents I know keep a bag of fresh-frozen vegetables on hand for those days when there's no time to warm up a meal. Babies who are nine months or more love to play with the thawed little morsels and feel the new textures in their mouths, even though the peas usually come out whole in their diapers. In fact, many favorite finger foods, such as beans, blueberries, and other fibrous items, aren't completely digested by babies under two years old.

Combinations are a great way to introduce a new food that baby may not be crazy about. Simply add more and more of the new flavor until it's a familiar taste. I got really carried away with such mixtures for our first daughter. One of our favorite baby pictures shows her grimacing after being fed a big bite of plain yogurt and mashed chicken liver!

I find it easier to hand a baby crusts of whole grain toast than to spoon cereal into her mouth. If you rely on table foods from the beginning, your baby won't face a transition from strained foods to chunkier mixtures.

After toast, she's ready to tackle bits of whole grain pasta, and then it's on to spaghetti and casseroles. (You'll discover that a baby who's just eaten spaghetti and then bathed will leave an orange ring around the tub!)

## Avoiding A Sweet Tooth

According to Dr. Lendon Smith, a baby's first foods influence her lifelong eating habits. "It's important not to start her on a lifelong love affair with sweet tastes by getting her used to sweet stuff," he advises.

The natural sugars found in fruit, vegetables, grains, and breastmilk are perfect for our bodies. But any other added sweeteners, including natural sweeteners but especially refined sugar and the new synthetic brands, crowd out other foods we really need.

You've probably seen babies being given sips of soda, or bites from a doughnut; not only are they developing a taste for sweets, but their stomachs are filling up with empty calories instead of valuable vitamins and minerals. Your baby's stomach is about the size of her fist, and should be filled with breastmilk and other ideal foods. She has the rest of her life to develop a sweet tooth on her own, so don't get her started on one now.

# Don't Offer Until the First Birthday. . .

Though your baby will love most foods before he's a year old, there are some you should hold off on. Raw honey, for example, shouldn't be given to a child under a year of age (he may get botulism from it), and foods such as whole hot dogs, peanuts, popcorn, and grapes can cause choking in any child under the age of four.

Your child may be spared some food sensitivities if you don't serve him egg white or cow's milk until he's about a year old. He's already getting his milk from you, and doesn't need the calories or butterfat. If your baby prefers soft textures, moisten food with breast-milk or water.

**If your family has a history of allergies, be slow to offer pork, fish, nuts, cabbage, corn, tomatoes, citrus juice, onions, wheat, rye, yeast, chocolate, and all berries. While most babies won't have a problem, some need to wait a while.**

Hold off on raw vegetables, except for a bit of grated carrot, until your baby has enough teeth to handle stringy celery or brittle zucchini. While a teething baby may love to chomp on a chilled carrot stick, his new teeth can break it into small bits that are easy to choke on. Wait until after the first year to introduce strawberries and citrus. Also abstain from condiments, such as catsup, mayonnaise, salt, and pepper.

**Food for Thought.** But try *not* to shield him from foods you dislike. Babies often devour foods we don't expect them to like. If we cheerfully serve them wholesome vegetables, beans, and whole grains, they'll probably retain a taste for them. We will also save ourselves from forever preparing special foods for finicky family members. Kids won't develop a taste for tomato and cheese sandwiches if they've only had peanut butter and jelly. ■

Now you're seeing the rewards of feeding your baby your own food. He's a happy family member who enjoys his meals with gusto!

# Extra Liquids

Of course, breastmilk should still be your baby's main liquid. And now that he's eating other foods, he's also getting moisture from fruits and vegetables. Thus you can hold off from offering extra liquids.

Nutritionally speaking, it's much better to eat a whole, vitamin- and fiber-rich orange or apple than drink its juice, especially since fruit juice has often been boiled and diluted with water. Many nutritionists recommend that liquids not be served at meals so that a child can fill up on foods rather than drinks.

## Mastering the Cup

Perhaps your baby is swiping at cups and desperately trying to drink from bowls, plates, and anything else with a drop of something still in it. (Our son was partial to the cat's water dish, while another little boy tried to suck water out of the garden hose.) He probably doesn't need extra liquids. But he may be ready to master a new skill and take another step toward independence. Drinking from a cup is a stage of weaning, and you'll be able to avoid bottles by allowing your baby to drink by himself as he gets older. You'll prevent the problem of the bottle becoming too much of a toy or pacifier if your child learns to use a cup.

Once your baby is well-established with solid foods, buy a small, unbreakable cup and let him play with it. Your local market probably has several varieties of baby cups, usually with handles and plastic tops, perhaps weighted at the bottom.

As your baby gets older, he'll use the handles to fling the cup across the room. He'll soon become skilled at taking off the top and pouring juice everywhere, so you may want to leave off the top entirely. For now, let him play with a cupful of water a few times each day. You'll see some sputtering as he occasionally hits himself with a faceful!

It will be several weeks before your drinker is actually swallowing much. When he does begin to swallow, you might feel brave enough to give him a quarter-inch or so of unsweetened fruit or vegetable juice, checking for any allergic reactions.

# Juice: Enjoy in Moderation!

Several experts warn against relying too much on fruit juice for our liquid intake. A child who drinks too much sweet juice may grow up to have an underslung jaw from not chewing enough. And juice is not as nutritious as eating the solid fruit.

Apple juice is a beginner's favorite, and you can also offer juices from foods he's already eating. Many older babies love carrot juice, as well as mixed tastes such as apple-berry juices.

As with other foods, juice that's as fresh as possible is the most wholesome and flavorful. Take a taste-test yourself: sip some fresh-squeezed orange juice and compare it to the type made from frozen concentrate. Apple juice loses quite a bit of taste and nutrition once it's been pasteurized and bottled.

**In general, you're better off drinking water than transparent juice, since most of the food value has been lost in juice and you're mainly getting a sweet taste.**

Read the labels of canned juices. Juice labeling can be tremendously deceiving: some cans or boxes on your supermarket shelves contain a mere ten percent pure juice. The label *must* say 100% pure, unsweetened juice for it to be the real thing!

**Food for Thought.** Now that your baby is flinging cups and moving about, it's time to child-proof your house. The kitchen is the best place to begin:

- Wind up all long electric cords; children love to pull on something to see it come down.

- Put up all houseplants, since some are poisonous when eaten or rubbed on the skin.

- Keep kitchen tools and supplies (cleaners, foil, plastic wrap) out of sight and out of reach. Potentially harmful kitchen items include insect sprays, drain cleaner, vitamins, and furniture polish.

- Let your child watch you cook, but don't place a highchair too close to the counter.

- Keep an eye on whatever goes in your toddler's mouth, especially small, easy-to-choke-on foods or toys. Even a child who can hold her own bottle must be watched.

- If your teething toddler has been given a numbing topical anesthetic, she may not be able to swallow some solid foods, so watch her carefully.

- All food must be well-cooked and cut into tiny pieces. ∎

# Food Allergies and Sensitivities: Tips for All Ages

Once you introduce solids, your child will be eating foods that aren't as easy to digest as breastmilk. "Mother's milk is one hundred percent pure as far as being metabolized and absorbed," says Dr. Joyce Virtue. "But other foods can trigger allergies, depending on a family's history and if the food is eaten too much and too often."

Such reactions may suddenly crop up in a six-month-old as well as a sixty-year-old, often from similar foods. The symptoms of allergic children can be few or many: puffy face, nasal stuffiness, asthmatic cough, hives, rash, and irritability.

You may also see "allergic shiners," which look like black eyes, or an "allergic salute" as a child constantly rubs his scratchy, runny nose. During one summer vacation of unfamiliar food and weather, one of our daughters developed a light-colored wrinkle across the bridge of her nose from itching it so much.

Your child may be allergic to her wool blanket or to carpet dust, or perhaps she just has a summer cold. An irritable baby may have an allergy, or may be frustrated by an ear infection, vision problems, or pinworms (a common childhood infestation of tiny white worms which live in intestines but come out at night to lay their eggs around the anus). But if your baby is fussy just after eating a new solid, or if your two-year-old has a sore bottom after eating strawberries, you're probably seeing a food sensitivity or allergy.

A true allergy is the body's reaction to a certain substance that has been inhaled, eaten, or touched. Once the allergen is detected, our bodies make countless antibodies that attack the offender and then remain dormant until a recurrence.

My husband, for instance, has a violent reaction to long-hair cats. His reserve of antibodies, while attacking the allergen, also releases chemicals (such as histamine) which cause his eyes to puff up and his nose to become stuffy. Left in the same room with a cat, he finds life miserable. Yet soon after the cat is removed, his symptoms disappear.

Food allergies work the same way. Some children may be allergic to milk if their mothers drank too much of it during pregnancy. They may swallow lots of milk because they crave the calcium, according to Dr. Smith, yet their intestines are actually rejecting the milk because of the allergy.

Cow's milk seems to be the greatest allergen if given before the age of twelve months, especially among formula-fed babies who aren't able to digest such foreign protein. If your baby isn't totally breastfed, ask your doctor about substitutes.

Fortunately, breastmilk is a familiar and perfect food, especially for allergic babies, because it contains immunological factors which protect against allergens.

## When To Consider Testing

If you suspect that your child has a food sensitivity or allergy, you may want to contact your pediatrician for a physical exam and advice on home detection, especially if your child is taking medication or experiencing breathing difficulties. There are several methods for laboratory allergy testing, including the popular skin test, and some tests may be better for children than adults.

"Personally, I hate to see a skin test done on a child," says Dr. Joyce Virtue. "It takes so long, is very painful, and is good for testing pollen allergies but not good for foods. Instead, I prefer a blood test (enzyme-linked amino acid test), which is more dependable for food allergies."

**Dr. Virtue and other experts feel that testing may also be helpful in detecting other suspected food reactions. Perhaps your child goes "off the wall" after taking that pink antibiotic for an ear infection: he could be reacting to its sugar, colorings, or to the drug itself.**

Luckily, many children outgrow food allergies. And you can quickly cleanse your young baby's system by totally breastfeeding him (an older child should eat a bland diet for several weeks). Then, watch for reactions (sore bottom, runny nose, etc.) as you re-introduce single foods. Ask your doctor about allergy testing methods you can safely do at home.

**Food for Thought.** Your child's skin rash or respiratory difficulty could also be caused by his environment. In Los Angeles, for example, burning, watery eyes and a hacking cough during bad bouts of air pollution are sad facts of life. Short of moving far away to a place with lots of fresh air, we're stuck with breathing hydrocarbons, ozone, particulates, and all the rest of it. One defense against such pollutants is an antioxidant supplement with combinations of vitamins A, C, E, and certain B vitamins, according to Dr. Virtue.■

Here are some of the most common allergens: tomatoes, citrus fruits, onions, chocolate, any drinks with caffeine, medications, vitamins, and fluoride. Keep in mind that children often outgrow allergies, so you can casually re-introduce a food as your child grows older.

Many families also avoid the repercussions of allergies by following a "rotation" diet which keeps them out of the rut of eating the same foods or food groups every day. Ask your pediatrician about ways to best tailor your family's diet in case of allergies. "There's no doubt that we'd be seeing less allergies if people didn't eat one food too much and too often," says Dr. Lendon Smith.

Try devising four or five favorite breakfast menus that you can alternate regularly. For lunch and dinner, choose widely among the food groups. Have whole wheat bread at the dinner table one night, brown rice the next, perhaps a barley dish the third. You'll widen your tastes and culinary horizons, and eat more wisely while you're at it.

Susan Harnett, co-owner of the "Bread and Circus" natural foods markets in Boston, is one parent who's felt the thrill of successful allergy testing. "Since we discovered that our son was reacting to unfamiliar foods, we now know why family trips were often stressful. It wasn't that he hated to travel; he was reacting to all the food we don't eat at home!"

It is true that what we eat can control our behavior. Thanks to the attention and care you give in selecting her food to grow on, your child will be her brightest, happiest self!

# FUN IN THE KITCHEN WITH YOUR
# SOCIABLE SIX-MONTH-OLD

*Some great six-month recipes in the back of this book:*

Applesauce Whip

Delicious Mush

Fruit Juice Finger Food

Journeycakes

Potato Pancakes

Vegetable Pancakes

Zucchini Cakes

# 4 THE YEAR-OLD NATURAL GOURMET

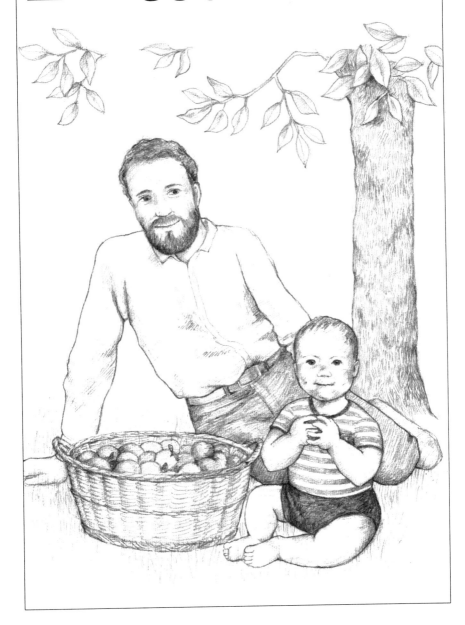

## Between One and Two Years of Age, Your Child May

- know many words and form two-word sentences

- walk, climb, and run without help

- begin to imitate you in scribbling, cooking, and household activities

- mimic you in brushing his teeth (a little toothpaste on his very own brush is delightful), but you need to brush his teeth after food is eaten until he is at least six

- love to look at a picture book, and anticipate a bedtime story

**H**APPY BIRTHDAY! Your one-year-old is probably dashing all over the place, either at a reckless crawl or a wobbly run. You'd think that all this activity would make her ravenous, burning up as much food as you can hand her, right?

Not usually. Walking babies seem to forget about eating once they're off in search of bigger and better adventures. Once content to sit in a highchair and play with peas, they're now wise to the fact that the world is an exciting place.

**It will be years before your child has a substantial attention span or appetite. If she clamors to get down after five minutes of nibbling, ask her if she's done and let her go!**

Heaven knows it's hard to resist coaxing her to take "just one more bite." But kids know when not to overeat. You don't want to hear her lament someday, "I'm not overeating. I'm just over-served."

# What To Feed Your Toddler

Her food needs are minimal: several servings a day of each food group, offered at mealtimes or snacks offered throughout the day. A great dinner for your one-year-old can be a small cube of cheese or meat, ten peas, a few bites of boiled potato, two ounces of juice, and perhaps some banana for dessert. Not exactly a feast by our standards, but just right for her tiny stomach. Try to follow these daily guidelines:

**Three servings** from the milk and cheese group, such as ½ cup of milk, plain yogurt, or custard. Many toddlers love to walk around with their own small bowl of grated cheese; about ¾ ounce is plenty.

**Four servings** from the fruit and vegetable group, such as two ounces of unsweetened juice, about three tablespoons lightly steamed dark green or yellow vegetables, plus a raw food such as banana, apple, or carrot. Offer these foods as snacks, and let your toddler help make a salad!

**Four servings** from the whole grain bread and cereal group, such as ½ slice of bread, ¼ cup unsweetened dry or cooked cereal, and ¼ cup pasta or rice. These selections are easy to offer and to fortify with extra peanut butter, fruit, or cream sauce.

**Two servings** of high quality protein, such as two tablespoons of peanut butter on whole grain bread, or one egg stirred into cereal as it cooks. Two tablespoons of lean, cooked meat can be cut into toddler-sized bites. You can also offer some cooked, dried peas or beans along with her rice to give her a complete protein.

## Appealing to Tiny Appetites

To entice little tastebuds when all his favorite meals have become old hat, offer more "grown-up" finger fare. Cooked carrots, for instance, are appealing when served in rows, and calling broccoli "green trees" makes it a funny food. Slice fruits and vegetables into rings, and use cookie cutters on bread. Use twisty pasta instead of straight spaghetti. Let him pour water from a toy teapot or plastic measuring cup into his own tiny cup at "teatime."

If you suspect teething misery, offer cold treats such as frozen custard, juice popsicles, or fruit milk (fresh fruit, ice, and a splash of milk whirled in a blender). Such good appetizing treats, served with a smile, make mealtimes a fun surprise!

**Food for Thought.** Talk with your pediatrician about vitamin supplements for your one-year-old. "Calcium, magnesium, and the B vitamins are often a main deficiency," says Dr. Lendon Smith. Your toddler will also be strengthened if vitamin C is slipped into his juice. If you'd like to fortify your cooking, add dashes of wheat germ, dolomite, kelp, and brewer's yeast. Just be sure any supplements are free of additives and sugar. It's crucial that our children get enough nutrients, since a child's brain has at least twice the energy needs of an adult's. Even with the best food to grow on, your child may need an additional boost. ■

An older baby may fall into a food hang-up, so serve new tastes at the beginning of a meal when she's hungriest. Our older daughter requested yogurt constantly for about a month when she was fifteen months old. By giving her a small cup of yogurt at snacktime and a variety of new foods when she was especially hungry at meals, she didn't forget about the foods she had liked before.

If you introduce strawberries, citrus, and other allergens, do so with caution. Whole cow's milk can be enjoyed from a cup now and then if there are no reactions. Just remember that solid foods take priority over liquids.

In fact, your toddler has enough teeth and coordination to handle most all but heavily salted, sweetened, and spicy dishes. Ignore nuts and seeds for another year or so; use nut butters instead. Skip whole hot dogs, grapes, and other foods which are more than an inch in diameter and too easily swallowed whole.

Baby food bottles, jars, and cans can be phased out completely. By now, your "big girl" is probably climbing up to take her own place at the table. Give her a spoon of her own and she'll sharpen her coordination, even though proficiency won't come until she's about two years old. Toddlers seem to alternate continuously between gobbling their food and playing with it.

**Between meals, let your toddler help herself to cut-up raw vegetables and fruit. You can keep a special "goodie" plate in the refrigerator within her reach. Set out some cheese and whole grain crackers with peanut butter to thwart the "four o'clock grouchies."**

Your toddler will slim down and gain only about four pounds by the time he's two, a big change from more than doubling his birth weight last year. Says Dr. Smith, "As long as he's laughing more than crying, don't worry about him not eating enough. The best approach is to offer only the most nourishing, best foods you can provide!"

**Food for Thought.** There's nothing like a tantrum-prone toddler to remind us that we all have a stubborn streak: for every "no" we hand out, we get at least two in return. Children need loving guidance more than the seemingly inevitable stream of "no-no's" they soon become accustomed to. If we try to treat them as *learning* rather than "naughty" creatures, and show them with patience, hugs, and kisses that we understand their frustrations, our attitude will carry over to the food we eat. Lecturing, spanking, and slapping have no place at the dinner table (or elsewhere), and only create a fear of punishment which transforms into a hatred of mealtimes. Because meals play a major part in our lives, we should offer our children their food to grow on with the same love we would bestow at gift-giving time. After all, good food and good health are two of the greatest gifts we can give. ∎

# Cooking With Your One-Year-Old

I think children are born wanting to help. Certainly by the time they're walking, they *need* to push the vacuum cleaner, water the flowers, and help with anything else Mom and Dad are doing. Your child's strong desire to imitate is a real boon in teaching her to appreciate nutritious food. In fact, she is already learning about what's good to eat from what you serve her.

A kitchen is the warmest, friendliest place to be, whether you're a grown-up attending a party or a first-grader wanting to finish homework. If it's not already, your kitchen will soon become the hub of your house. For toddlers, it's the place nearest to their parents. And not only that, it's just full of new tools to master! A young child's thrill of feeding herself soon gives way to the pride of learning how to make her own food.

Give her raisins to decorate faces on oatmeal, to arrange "ants" on celery stalks stuffed with peanut butter or cream cheese, or to set "eyes" into a loaf of bread. Older toddlers like to use toothpicks to hold cheese cubes or rolled up meat slices.

With her own small plastic measuring cup, a child can pour milk over her own bowl of cereal, or juice into her cup. A one-year-old can sit on the counter and help stir pancake batter, then watch the pancakes turn brown on the griddle. Let her carry a pancake to the table by herself and deliver it to another family member. Not only will she devour those pancakes she helped create, but she'll learn how to give pleasure to other people.

Toddlers are terrific at making casseroles. They love to sample noodles, beans, or browned meat, and grated cheese that might have seemed "yucky" if they hadn't seen it being prepared. Let them help you make dinner in the mid-afternoon and they'll automatically get a great snack.

Kids of all ages love cookie cutters of assorted shapes. Show your child how to cut out roller cookies, or shapes from bread or toast for a fun sandwich. Give her a small piece of dough the next time you make bread. (Be prepared: even much older kids prefer to eat the dough rather than wait for it to be baked.) She'll be thrilled to see her own steaming, fragrant roll coming out of the oven!

## First Chores

A toddler can set the table by himself with unbreakable plates, cups, and utensils. He can even pull the napkins out of a low drawer and place one by each person's place. At the end of the meal, he can carry his cup to the sink, or perhaps wipe off the table with a sponge.

For the ultimate thrill, let your toddler help tear lettuce as you chop other vegetables for a salad. He can drop soup ingredients into a pot or bowl, and give the concoction a good stir before it goes on the stove.

If you're feeling adventurous, let your child break an egg into a bowl for scrambled eggs. This can be quite a slimy experience, but he'll soon learn how if you gently hold his hands over the egg and show him how to pull the cracked shell apart.

## Table Manners

Table manners for toddlers are minimal at best. In fact, toddler etiquette has peaked when there's just one food fight per day. I count my blessings when our son stays in his chair, doesn't drop too much food, and wipes his mouth with a napkin when we ask him to at the end of his meal. He can keep his cup upright most of the time, sometimes spear a carrot with a salad fork (the plastic ones are useless), and stay seated for about five minutes before climbing out of his chair.

He tries to imitate his sisters and join in the conversation, especially when mealtime is cheerful and pleasant. Asking him to do much more would be unfair, so we simply wait for the time when his abilities improve enough for him to follow his family's example of good manners. By the time he's two-and-a-half, he'll actually prefer a fork over his fingers most of the time.

Take heart and relax, since your child's atrocious table manners will improve as his coordination and attention increase. Smile at his small accomplishments and he will sense your approval as he slowly masters the spoon and fork, or keeps his food within a reasonable distance of his plate.

The mere idea of trying to monitor the social graces of a toddler at the table makes me tense, and I don't want to communicate tension across the table to my child. No matter how attractive his food, he will (like all toddlers) act up in any situation that is not accepting and warm.

# Kitchen Safety

Along with his new kitchen skills, your toddler will need to learn about the prime kitchen hazards: heat, glass, sharp edges, electrical outlets, and moving parts.

There are two schools of thought about children helping in the kitchen: they should be forbidden to touch the stove until they can read the dials, or they should learn as early as possible about respecting the stove and other dangers.

I favor the latter approach, as long as the parent keeps an extremely watchful eye and doesn't slack off for years. Our seven-year-old can read a recipe and assemble and measure ingredients. Our five-year-old is adept at using pot holders and removing a cake pan from the oven, while her year-old brother can set the kitchen timer (but not to any special time), put forks on the table, and punch the oven light to check how the cake is baking.

His stirring, sifting, pounding, and tasting are limited to the kitchen table or a place at the counter away from the range burners. Yet if I'm standing right there, he's welcome to sit on the counter near the heat and watch the soup bubble or the sauce thicken. He already knows the meaning of "hot" by testing the food I've put on his plate, and he's touched some warm pans (while I've watched) to learn for himself that he can't handle everything in the kitchen.

By the time he's three, he'll be familiar enough with heat to stir a pudding until it boils. He'll also probably have the coordination and logic to hold an electric beater with one hand and the handle of a bowl with the other (as an adult stands by).

## Good Cooking Habits

Just as your child's lifelong eating habits are shaped by the food you give him, so are his cooking habits. A child who knows how to fix a whole wheat pizza with his favorite fresh toppings will be less likely to crave a microwave version with fake ingredients. Likewise, a teenager who knows how to cook whole foods will be accustomed to their taste and more receptive to natural fare.

These predictions might seem like future-gazing to you as you read them and then glance at your toddler. You're already well on your way towards building a better future as your child learns how to enjoy and create whole food family favorites.

# We Are What We Eat . . .

Now that your toddler enjoys a wider variety of food to grow on, you face some crucial questions about nutrition. He'll be exposed to more processed food, and you'll have to decide where to draw the line about fats, sweets, and junk. (See section on peer pressure in "Heading Off To School" chapter for more tips.)

It's easy to keep your toddler out of fast-food restaurants. A toddler would not know to ask for a Whopper, after all. And babies are not born with a craving for cola or sugar cereals!

**Food for Thought.** On the other hand, now might be the perfect time to see just how much your toddler is absorbing from the family TV. In this age of cable and cartoons, parents may soon hear "She-ra" and "Big Mac" as their baby's first words! Fast food and other industries spend mega-bucks to direct ads right at your child, so be careful what she watches. Often, she's instructed to *demand* certain products for her free toy giveaway or club offer. Some families make it a rule not to buy anything advertised on TV, and many talk about each ad with their older children. For a more radical approach, read *Four Arguments For the Elimination of Television* by Jerry Mander. Not only should we question the propaganda aimed at our children, but how does TV alter our imagination and ability to create images in our brains? ■

## Our Natural Love of Sweets

The sweetness of natural milk and fruits is accompanied by naturally occurring vitamins, minerals, and other nutrients. Sugar-laden candy, cookies, and cereals, on the other hand, pose a double-pronged threat: not only do some cereals contain more sugar than milk chocolate, but a child given such low-nutrition stuff learns to crave sugar and perhaps pursue it for the rest of his life.

> **Sugar is a simple carbohydrate that gives us fat deposits without the bonus of any vitamins, minerals, and other redeeming components. Some experts believe that sugar can be addicting and cause adverse physical reactions, including hyperactivity and an inability to concentrate.**

Unlike natural foods, refined sugar is a devitalized food substance with no fiber attached. It's almost pure glucose, which zips into our systems quickly and displaces B vitamins, sending our blood sugar sky-high. Our body, sensing the overload, floods us with insulin to neutralize the glucose. The result is often a crashing depression and a craving for more sweets.

Probably the biggest problem with refined sweeteners is that they appear in most every packaged supermarket item, from vegetables to bread.

**Food for Thought.** Reducing sugar in your foods will also reduce many preservatives and other chemicals in your diet. (Few honey-sweetened cookies, for example, have had suspected carcinogens BHA or BHT added.) You may actually feel some withdrawal symptoms as you cut out a food you're addicted or allergic to. As you switch from sugar, cut it gradually from your recipes, and use whole grain flours in your baking to substitute for the texture stiffening function of sugar. By the way, white flour is so refined and denatured that our intestines treat it the same as sugar.■

It's not always easy to abandon sugar after years of using it. Some people gradually replace it with other sweeteners, and others quit all at once. You can begin by reducing the sweetening in your favorite recipes by one fourth without a significant difference in flavor and texture.

You have lots of other choices!

## A Primer on Sweeteners

The recipes in this book call for alternative sweeteners, such as honey, molasses, maple syrup, dried fruit, and fruit juice concentrates. If you don't want to give up cane sugar immediately, try to substitute one of these until you're well on the road away from relying on too many sweeteners in your meals.

**Honey** is a favorite white sugar replacement. Buy raw, unfiltered, and unheated honey. It's already sterile, so doesn't need to have its taste and nutritive values destroyed by pasteurization. Experiment with different flavors, since honey tastes like what the bees have been feeding upon. Kids love to compare orange or clover honey with the stronger flavor of avocado honey.

**Maple syrup** can be used for an even sweeter flavor. Buy the pure stuff, not the usual blends of corn syrup with a dash of fake maple flavoring and preservatives. Look for brands from Canada, since Canadian laws forbid the practice of injecting any formaldehyde into trees to increase the sap flow.

# Honey Hints

- 1 cup sugar = ¾ cup honey. Decrease other liquid by ½ cup, or add ¼ cup more flour per ¾ cup honey.

- For brown sugar flavor: equal parts honey/maple syrup or honey/light molasses

- For pancake topping: equal parts honey/molasses, warmed, with a dash of vanilla

**Molasses** comes in several varieties and flavors. Especially nutritious is blackstrap, a strong, dark by-product of sugar refining. For a lighter color and more delicate flavor, try unsulfured (Barbados) molasses. Molasses has traces of B vitamins, calcium, phosphorus, and iron.

**The above sticky sweeteners are much easier to use if you first measure your oil or butter, then use that cup to pour your honey or whatever.**

**Dried fruit** is another popular natural sweetener. (After all, how exciting is an oatmeal cookie without raisins?) Yet there are drawbacks: it's as much as 75 percent sugar and it sticks to teeth. Look at the ingredients list on packages, since dried fruit is often treated with preservatives or coloring agents. Ask for date pieces rolled in oat flour, or whirl unsweetened coconut in a blender to use as a white sugar replacement.

# Date Flour

Whirl equal portions of whole grain flour and date pieces in your blender. Substitute ½ cup date flour for each cup of white or wheat flour in recipes, and leave out sugar entirely.

**Fruit juice concentrates** are perhaps the best option to use in place of refined sugar, honey, or corn syrup. Buy cans of frozen, unsweetened juices and thaw them to use as sweeteners in your favorite recipes. Our favorite mixed fruit concentrate is a mixture of pure pineapple syrup, pear, and peach juice. Apple and pear juices are easy to use; substitute them for liquid and sugar in a recipe, and use baking soda instead of baking powder.

**Carob** is a chocolate substitute which, if unsweetened, is a nutritious, good-tasting ingredient in your baking. While one ounce of unsweetened chocolate needs a cup of sugar to make it edible, carob is naturally sweet and doesn't have the fat, calories, caffeine, and tannic acid of chocolate. Ask your store owner for unsweetened carob chips and powder, or see "Recommended Readings and Resources" for Sunlight Foods and other sources.

As you experiment with alternative sweeteners, you'll soon lose much of your obsession for sugary stuff. Rather than feeling a false hunger and craving an entire chocolate layer torte, you'll be satisfied with a smidgen of whole wheat spice cake. As Dr. Lendon Smith says, turning away from sugar is another way of learning how to "read our own bodies."

## Food for Thought.

Hyperactivity, defined as an inability to ignore unimportant stimuli, is estimated to affect up to ten percent of our school-age children. You may spot an abnormal restlessness in your child at a very early age; some babies show symptoms of frequent crib rocking and head knocking. Perhaps your child is in constant motion, dancing, running, and behaving in a way that seems beyond his control. While some physicians feel that there is no correlation between sugar or additives and our behavior, many advise us to alter our diets before trying drugs to curb hyperactivity. It's also important to know that a hyperactive child may be misdiagnosed. There's no one test for hyperactivity; indeed, "the diagnosis is one of simple observation," says Dr. Lendon Smith. Some overactive kids may be reacting to a lack of interesting, stimulating activities. Maybe their erratic behavior is a cry for attention, a plea often unanswered by a physician with "behavior controlling" drugs. To help their hyperactive youngsters, parents can create the best possible environment at home. Dr. Smith feels that some borderline-hyperactive children may respond with an excellent diet and perhaps supplements, such as calcium for stress, B vitamins for improved memory, or a pick-me-up protein snack. For more information about how diet affects behavior, read *Feed Your Kids Bright* by Francine and Harold Prince (1987, Simon and Schuster) and ask your doctor about recent findings about hyperactivity. ■

# When to Stop Nursing

You may be reading this with a six-month-old in your lap. Or perhaps you want to learn more about weaning a two-year-old. Some moms decide exactly when to cut off breastfeeding even before their baby arrives; others try to force extended nursing.

Both approaches are severe. Our society seems obsessed with the issue of when to cut off breastfeeding, yet in most cultures mothers nurse their young for *years* after birth. There are absolutely *no medical reasons* for an early weaning, even though some grandparents might swear that breastfeeding causes everything from obesity, tooth decay, homosexuality, and so on.

## Why Do You Want To Wean?

Ask yourself what it is that you and others want to achieve by weaning. Your independence? Increased self-sufficiency for your child? Freedom from the "embarrassment" of nursing? It might help to identify which of your concerns come from society's pressures and which come from your own goals for your child's nutrition and your special nursing relationship with him.

There are many excellent reasons to nurse your child until his first birthday, if not longer. First, your milk is still the most perfect food you can give him; the pass-through immunities, antibodies, and vitamins make it superior to any formula you can buy. Second, you're avoiding allergies by keeping him on the breast rather than introducing a new milk source.

Medical grounds aside, you're extending the close relationship you've shared since his birth. Maybe your baby is so active that nursing is the only time the two of you can be close, which makes it an even more perfect way to meet his needs.

As a newborn, he nursed for food as well as love. At six months, your milk is not his sole food source, yet it is still superb for his physical growth. And at a year, he may still want the security of his old relationship. Many moms with feverish toddlers have been thankful that their children were still nursing, not only as a means of nourishment but as a familiar comfort.

**Food for Thought.** When should you wean? No matter how persuasive the reasons to nurse, it's still up to you and your baby. Some moms "don't want to be pulled on" after the first three months, when they feel too tired and pestered to continue. Others have thought their babies self-weaned at nine months, only to discover that their child just needed a little extra encouragement. It's unusual for a baby to wean herself before the age of two, according to La Leche League co-founder Marian Thompson. Once you feel you are no longer enjoying nursing, it's time to stop; gradually, with love. The key to successful weaning is for it to be gentle, and accompanied by tender distractions. The older the child, the easier the weaning. ■

## Gentle Weaning

If you're weaning an infant, you'll need to find another food that's as similar to breastmilk as possible. Try to cancel one feeding every week or so; a gradual switch to bottles is much easier on both of you. Your baby won't feel cheated, you won't feel as guilty or emotional, and your breasts won't become engorged.

Talk to your doctor about supplements to fortify the formula. And don't yield to the temptation of propping up baby's bottle and going off to do something else; your baby needs just as much cuddling as when he nursed. Think of your embrace as a supplement of its own.

Older babies can be taken directly from the breast to the cup. When I weaned our oldest daughter, we bought some pretty new plastic cups and a small bottle of juice for her to enjoy when she became thirsty. Weaning to a cup is the ideal way to go, and such little tricks like the one we used can make it much easier.

**One mom told me, "I really regret substituting a bottle for nursing. My daughter wanted to cling to it and suck constantly, much more than when we nursed! And it was so much harder to get rid of that**

**bottle when she was older!" While a bottle might
provide a food replacement, it certainly can't replace *you*, so plan on spending extra time with your
baby in new ways.**

La Leche League offers this advice for gradually weaning a
child over six months: *"Don't offer, don't refuse."* As long as you
keep up her liquid intake through other means, you can wait for her
to ask before you pick her up to nurse. Although an older child is
more easily distracted, even a six-month-old can forget to nurse
now and then if she's eating food to grow on.

Once your child is a year old, you can rest easy about the
loss of breastmilk from a nutritional standpoint. Her varied diet of
whole foods is in place and her need for milk has decreased.

## Distracting the Older Baby

An active one-year-old usually nurses far less than a younger
baby does, often limiting her feeding sessions to once before a nap
and once upon waking. Perhaps she makes other requests out of
boredom or habit: you can distract her by reading to her, gardening
with her, or offering to let her help with housework.

You can easily anticipate the usual nursing requests. Does
your daughter ask to nurse when she sees you sitting down in a
favorite chair? Or does she always climb into your lap while you're
reading the paper? Try to distract her *before* she asks to nurse. Don't
sit down for a while, or choose a different place to read the paper.
Offer her a bit of fruit just as she wakes up from a nap, or let her
help you make dinner. Go for a walk. Wear a one-piece dress that
prohibits nursing. One friend told her son "All gone!" with a smile
and a laugh each time he approached her to nurse, then rough-
housed with him a bit for some physical closeness.

Any mother who weans her baby, no matter his age, can be
resourceful in discovering new ways to mother. While one parent
will be able to satisfy her child by reading and rocking him, another
will hand him an apple slice and declare that they're on their way to
the park. Our youngest daughter was especially partial to yogurt
popsicles. Such gentle diversions, over a few weeks or months, will
come close to "baby-led" weaning, with a little help from you.

**If you do decide to continue nursing, rest assured that your child will eventually stop. What now seem like marathon nursing sessions will shortly dwindle to nearly nothing. Many moms who have nursed beyond infancy had no intention of doing so: it simply happened!**

There are ways to make long-term nursing easier. I'm a big fan of nursing "etiquette," especially when others may take offense at breastfeeding. You might try teaching your toddler a code word if you don't want others to guess what he's talking about. (Be careful, though. Some moms have thought it cute to hear their one-year-old ask for "booby," and are later mortified to hear it in public.)

Luckily, the older child is blessed with a growing sense of patience. Since breastfeeding a toddler is often best done in private, you'll find yourself asking your child to wait. My year-old son recently asked to nurse while I was in the middle of a discussion with my daughters' principal. To him, it seemed the perfect time. I was sitting down, he was bored with all the office knick-knacks. . .

Needless to say, I distracted him. And he understood, especially since I promised to ask him later if he still wanted to nurse. (He usually doesn't.) If he had been truly thirsty, I would have given him the small box of juice I always carry in my purse for just such occasions.

Sometimes it isn't convenient or appropriate to nurse, even when he slinks down into position. In such a case, I'll just whisper "no, not now," and amuse him with a toy or point out another youngster. This tactic works about nine out of ten times, especially if I get up and move my position to afford him a more interesting view.

As in all areas of his life, a mobile child needs loving guidelines with nursing, eating, and the simpler manners. It's often a judgment call: your toddler may sometimes just be goofing around and not really need to nurse. Be creative as you try to fill his needs.

## Second Thoughts and Alternatives

Before you begin actively weaning, you should discuss with your mate the reasons why you want to stop breastfeeding. Are you exhausted? Weaning isn't going to help that much; you may spend more time preparing bottles and feeding them to your baby. Rather than nursing a sleepy baby in your warm bed, both of you will be wide-awake for a bottle feeding in the middle of the night. You might soon feel very sad and regret losing this special connection. Try to go to bed earlier, get some help around the house, or take a nightly hot bath.

Or perhaps you're uncomfortable with the idea of nursing a toddler. Find some friendly support in a neighborhood play group or a nursing mothers' support group. Ask other friends, parents you meet at the park, or your childbirth instructor about existing groups. You could start your own group, too. La Leche League often holds "Toddler Meetings" which focus on toddlers' special needs. Or call your local chapter for printed information about the benefits of extended breastfeeding; solid medical facts can be invaluable to both parents and friends of nursing toddlers.

Is your child perhaps using nursing as a way to get attention? Make sure you're giving him plenty of yourself. Distract him if you think he wants to nurse because he's bored, or examine your own lifestyle to see if he's feeling confused, lonely, or insecure.

I found that my younger daughter wanted to nurse whenever she saw me on the telephone. Since I was often conducting interviews, I'd pull her up on my lap and nurse her as a way to keep her quiet. Well, I got my work done, but the compromise certainly wasn't fully meeting her need for attention.

Once I started to make most of my phone calls during her naptime, she bounced back to her cheerful, confident self. Our nursing relationship continued until she simply forgot to nurse one day, and then another. About a month later, I realized that she'd moved on to new frontiers.

## Still Nursing and Pregnant?

You may find out while you're still nursing that you're pregnant. Some moms choose to wean gradually before they go to the hospital, while others wait a bit, and often find that their older baby has weaned himself. Many babies pick up on the fact that your milk supply has diminished. Others dislike the new taste, especially toward the end of pregnancy when colostrum replaces your milk.

Just remember to feel secure in continuing to nurse your toddler while you are pregnant. And be sure to eat a superior diet, which you'd want to do anyway. *If you are well-nourished, your nursing child will not steal calcium and vitamins from your unborn baby.* As a matter of fact, our second daughter was more than a pound-and-a-half heavier than our first child, who nursed throughout my pregnancy.

Nursing while pregnant helps toughen a mom's nipples, as well as preventing breast engorgement. As an added bonus, your older child won't feel abandoned once the new baby arrives. Tandem nursers are like twins. They often hold hands while they nurse, increasing their sense of warmth and love for each other.

Your new infant will be getting plenty of milk, and his older sibling won't feel kicked out of the nest. Your breasts will still produce enough to meet the demand. Remember, your toddler won't be nursing all that often, and you'll probably be able to distract him. Being able to nurse (or read to) your older child is a great way to feed the baby and keep track of your toddler at the same time! I also found it a great way to take an afternoon nap together during those few months after birth.

Again, listen to your own feelings on the issue of weaning. It's much better just to cuddle your child with all your love than to nurse begrudgingly, and any toddler will anxiously spot the difference between the two. Follow your heart. As long as you're both enjoying life together, wonderful!

# FUN IN THE KITCHEN WITH YOUR ONE-YEAR-OLD

- Pull down the dishwasher door to use as a table (our son loves to stir water in a bowl while I cook).

- Have one low shelf for "his" pots and pans, rubber bowls, and other unbreakable items.

- A *child's cooking supplies* can include empty yogurt containers, a set of plastic measuring spoons, an old wooden spoon, a plastic measuring cup, plastic cookie cutters, a funnel, and a rolling pin, a small vegetable scrubber brush, a tiny squeezable bottle of liquid soap.

- He can see what you're doing if he stands on his own sturdy barstool or chair at the counter.

- Or he can watch from his highchair and sample!

Once you have a toddler, nearly all your meals should be as quick and easy as possible. Don't be surprised if your baby gets hungry as he smells your dinner cooking and wants to help! Check the index for casserole recipes which you can double, freezing one of them to use on some future day.

*Recipes to spellbind tiny appetites:*

Barbecued Corn-on-
  the-Cob
Cheese Cookies
Cottage Cheese-Yogurt
  Pancakes
Drugstore Egg Custard

Gooey Chicken
Peach Cobbler
Pumpkin Pot Stew
Quick Fruit Ice Cream
Tuna Patties

# 5

# GROWING UP:

*Preschool Delights*

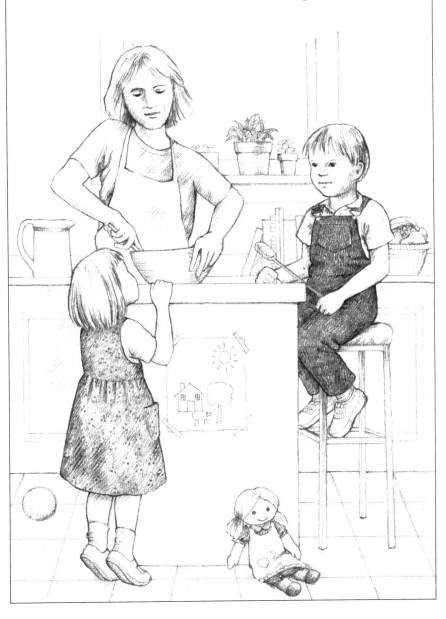

THE DAYS of independence are here. Your preschooler is officially a KID with more questions, stubborn streaks, and personality quirks than many adults you know! While you once spent hours diapering and nursing him, now he demands even more attention, and in new ways. Feeding him is no longer as simple as nursing or spooning in a few solid foods. It's often more a matter of supervision than nourishment.

After all, a preschooler isn't experienced enough to know which foods are the ones to grow on. All he knows is what tastes, looks, and feels appealing.

He'll be more interested in good foods if he's had a hand in their creation, so continue to invite him to cook with you. Cooking together is a great way to give preschoolers the attention, independence, and accomplishments they crave.

Maybe there's a new sibling demanding your attention, so your older child craves more time with you. If so, give him his own responsibilities: let him serve cereal or break up green beans.

Little changes can help your child become more self-reliant. Put a stool and cups in the bathroom and kitchen so he can satisfy his own thirst. Keep a plate of raw vegetables or other snacks on a low shelf in the refrigerator so he won't have to run to you every time he's hungry. In other words, try to give him new opportunities to grow up on his own terms.

# What to Feed Your Preschooler

Your active child can eat the same basic whole foods you do, except in smaller amounts. He should still be allowed to "graze" (especially on fresh fruits, vegetables, and protein foods like peanut butter, cheese, and eggs) to keep him from getting hungry and out-of-sorts.

In fact, the traditional "three square meals a day" approach is unnatural for most young people, who follow their inner instincts about food. Your child may not be gaining many pounds and inches each year, yet his language, intellectual, social, and physical skills are skyrocketing.

---

## Guidelines for Daily Preschooler Meals

*(Don't fret about fulfilling nutritional requirements. Just because your child is served an ideal diet doesn't mean that he needs every bite of it every day. Simply offer him a variety of food to grow on!)*

**Three servings** from the milk and cheese group, such as ½ cup milk, 1 ounce cheese, ½ cup yogurt, ¾ cup soup or pudding made with milk.

**Four servings** from the fruit and vegetable group, such as 2 tablespoons cooked vegetables, ½ cup fruit or unsweetened juice, ½ - 1 whole apple, orange, banana, tomato, or carrot.

**Four servings** from the whole grain bread and cereal group, such as ½ cup dry or cooked unsweetened cereal, 1 slice bread, ½ cup rice or pasta.

**Two servings** from the protein group, such as 2 tablespoons peanut butter, 1 egg, 3 tablespoons cooked, dried peas or beans, 3 tablespoons lean cooked meat, boneless fish, or poultry.

---

Aim for at least one good daily source of vitamin C. Strawberries, tomatoes, cabbage, and broccoli can be alternated with the more familiar citrus fruits and juices. Also get in the vitamin A habit: serve a dark green or yellow vegetable or fruit, such as carrots, dark green leafy vegetables, sweet potatoes, and winter squash at least every other day. If you're into calorie counting, your child needs about 1200 a day, increasing by 200 calories each year until the age of seven.

Babies' tiny stomachs can't hold much at one sitting, often not more than a quarter cup of peas, a bit of whole grain bread, and a few bites of other nutritious foods. With such a small appetite, your preschooler needs a wide variety of food to grow on, rather than a fluffy white roll that fills her up.

You can follow the same guidelines you used when she was a toddler, but serve more of each item. Offer wholesome treats throughout the day, let her natural growing spurts dictate her appetite, and continue to make mealtimes joyful.

## Perking Up Picky Eaters

You can nearly always single out the voice of a preschooler's parent: "He just won't eat a thing!" or, "She eats just like a bird!" The ages two through four are the infamous ages of "eating strikes," as kids temporarily slow down in their physical growth and seem to concentrate on mental leaps. They honestly don't need much food if they are between growth spurts, so don't worry about your finicky eater.

We have three children who are always in very different growing stages. They share the same food at each meal, and choose among several snack choices between meals. Here is a sample of the differing amounts of food they eat.

## SAMPLE OF FOOD INTAKE AT DIFFERENT AGES

| | Girl, 7 | Girl, 5 | Boy, 1 |
|---|---|---|---|
| *Breakfast:* | | | |
| French toast | 2 pieces | 1 piece | 1 piece |
| Eggs | 1 | 2 | ½ |
| Cantaloupe | 3 slices | ½ slice | 2 slices |
| Orange juice | 1 cup | 2 cups | ¼ cup |
| *Lunch:* | | | |
| Bologna sandwich with tomato | 1 | ½ | ½ |
| Cottage cheese | ½ cup | 2 cups | ¼ cup |
| Plum | 1 | ½ | 2 |
| Apple juice | ½ cup | 1 cup | ½ cup |
| *Dinner:* | | | |
| Baked chicken | 2 cups | 1 cup | 2 cups |
| Green salad | 2 cups | ½ cup | ¼ cup |
| Baked potato | 1 | ¼ | ½ |
| Slice of berry pie | 2 | 1 | 1 |
| Milk | ½ cup | 1 cup | ½ cup |

A glance at this chart tells me that our older daughter and our son are in growth spurts because they are eating a measurable amount of food more than they did last week. Our five-year-old, on the other hand, picks at her food and prefers to drink a lot of juice. Tomorrow I will pour her a small amount of juice and remove the juice container from the table so she'll concentrate on solid food.

And I won't draw attention to the fact that her little brother often eats more than she does. Within a few days she may dramatically announce starvation and gobble down an apple, two slices of raisin bread, and a carton of yogurt for a mid-morning snack, then move on to a hefty lunch.

Just for fun, try charting a day's worth of your child's food (but only if you can keep from worrying or conveying any anxiety to him about how much food he eats). Wait a week or two, and sooner or later he'll turn ravenous overnight, from hating bananas to eating two at once (or three if you set out a bowl of peanut butter for dipping).

Always be on the lookout for new ways to supply vital nutrients. If your child currently despises green vegetables, for example, serve just a smidgen of them and offer other foods with the same vitamins and minerals. A peach, for instance, is as nutritious as many vegetables, and few children will turn one away. Sometimes all that's needed is a bit of creativity.

---

## Fresh Fruit and Vegetable Creations

- Circular sandwich bites, such as cucumber or carrot rounds, between two cheese circles; or peanut butter spread between thin apple slices

- Peas or string beans right from the pod; kids love to open up anything hiding a treasure

- Chilled carrot curls or carrot sticks arranged like your kids' initials

- A fruit plate face, with a smile of cantaloupe, orange segment eyes, a strawberry nose, and coconut hair

- Cherry tomatoes stuffed with cottage cheese and parsley hair

---

Meals can really take on pizazz if you try foreign dishes and talk about the countries they come from. Our kids love to build their own tacos, pizzas, and sandwiches of pita bread. Even combined vegetables (usually their carrots and broccoli *must* remain isolated on opposite sides of the plate) quickly disappear if the kids have helped chop them up.

Another fun idea comes from the Swedes, who use a flat piece of bread as a plate for other foods. *Smorgasbord* means "sandwich board," and is a great way to give your preschooler a portable dinner. According to Viking tradition, food is selected and placed on the bread from a buffet arranged in this order: cold vegetables, cold fish dishes, cold meat, hot dishes such as meatballs, and desserts. Our kids prefer to eat each layer separately and save the bread for last.

For a Basque adventure, try a "family style" meal. An individual dish is passed around the table and everybody takes just what he wants. Each course is eaten entirely before the next bowl is passed. First pass fish or another appetizer. Then soup, followed by meat, green or yellow vegetables, and potatoes. You can let your child play for a spell between courses. Such a dinner is quite a change from our style of heaping our plates and eating quickly! And it's a creative way to start your preschooler on the road to making his own decisions.

## Other Ideas to Brighten Small Appetites

- Take your time. Get up half an hour earlier than usual for a relaxed breakfast. If your child has been playing hard, let her play quietly for about ten minutes before eating. Or serve dinner after your child hops out of a warm bath. If the dinner hour is late, feed her before the adults eat, and let her join you for fruit or dessert. (But don't get in the habit of watching her eat all alone. Meals are a lot more fun and relaxed with company.)

- Put some sparkle in everyday fare. Make a berry face on cereal, and she can pour her own milk from a cream pitcher or plastic measuring cup. (See ideas throughout this chapter on making meals more fun.)

- Make it small. Make it easy. And make it count. Put child-size portions on a favorite saucer: a bit of broccoli, a dollop of applesauce, and a cheese sandwich cut with a heart-shaped cookie cutter. A preschooler can be discouraged by mounds of food, so start off small and she'll ask for more if she wants any. Make it easy for her to feed herself. Our youngest daughter would never eat soups because "they slide off a spoon." I began offering either a thick, creamy soup, or letting her drink from the bowl.

- Keep conversation away from food, manners, and adult problems. Some kids are so sensitive to tension that their stomachs cramp, making eating impossible. I know one little girl who loses her appetite at the mere mention of homework. Instead, make mealtimes a chance for family togetherness.

## Playing Down Food Quirks

Of course, life isn't always easy just because our food is good. I recently about blew my top when all three kids refused to eat the food as I'd served it. One child whined because her enchilada was too big, her sister pouted when the refried beans on her plate touched the rice, and their brother only wanted to eat whatever was on the floor.

Such quirks used to drive me nuts, until a more mellow parent advised me to *treat my family as dinner guests* more often. So now, while our younger daughter gets a smaller plate for her tiny servings, our older needs a big plate "so all the food can breathe." Their younger brother prefers anything if it's on somebody else's plate. But don't go overboard in trying to cater to every whim. While I don't mind serving food on different sized plates, I draw the line at cooking different foods for each child.

The most popular meals are probably the simplest. As our daughter used to say, "I like my food just right. Not too hot, not too big, and not mixed up." (These words of wisdom were offered after she spurned a large, steaming portion of my favorite casserole.)

The result: she helped herself to some crunchy raw carrots, creamy cottage cheese, and whole wheat bread smeared with peanut butter and decorated with raisins. And I learned to serve smaller portions and let her food cool down so she could start eating right away. Not too much to ask, was it?

If your child enters a similar stage of pickiness, ask yourself how important the issue will be five years from now. For instance, will she suffer nutritionally or socially if she temporarily refuses to eat bread crusts?

If you feel strongly about wasting crusts, ask her how to solve the problem. Maybe those crusts could feed neighborhood birds, or go into a delicious bread pudding. (Let her be responsible for putting her crusts in a plastic bag for freezing.) She'll get an ego boost, and you'll have cut down on the number of rules everybody has to remember.

Part of her rebellion may also be a test to learn how to get what she wants, and to find out whether you'll nag or scold. Don't start the vicious cycle of fighting over food, or you'll run the risk of turning mealtimes into battle times. As your kids get older, you'll want to save your energy for more important issues than whether they finish their meals or not.

If your child doesn't want to eat any dinner, she should still sit at the table with you and talk about pleasant subjects. If the food remains untouched, kindly let her know that nothing will be offered until the next snack or meal, and simply clear the table.

One mom asked me, "How in the world did I start this game of yelling when she won't eat enough squash? Or rewarding her for eating a good meal?"

## Rewards

One of the most tempting traps of parenthood is the urge to reward our children for eating as much as we think they should. It's as if we still think kids in other countries will starve if we don't clean our plates. Actually, your child is in tune with his body, and you need to pay attention to his instincts. Given free rein with healthy foods, kids eat *to appetite*, neither over nor under their needs.

In particular, try to avoid the habit of rewarding with sweets. The parent who rewards a child with candy or ice cream isn't actually performing an act of love. After all, heart disease can begin very early in life. Besides, children would much rather be rewarded with your attention. Snuggle together with a book rather than just offering a candy bar. Or promise a trip to the park or zoo next weekend.

Food rewards give nutrition the wrong emphasis and can easily become a child's manipulating tool. I've talked with many parents who rue the day they used sweets as bribes for good manners, a better report card, toilet training, and so on.

"At first, my daughter would eagerly run to the toilet to get a chocolate kiss," says one dad. "But then the novelty wore off, and she realized we had a great big bag of candy in the kitchen. She started pretending to go to the bathroom every five minutes to keep up a steady stream of candy, then demanded two pieces for each attempt! My wife and I wonder why we started this business in the first place. We don't usually have candy in our house at all!"

Rather than reinforcing correct behavior, such rewards tell a child that junk food is better than healthy food, as well as more scarce and therefore more valuable. To a preschooler, the message is confusing: candy is usually not around because it isn't good for you, but if you make your parents happy, they'll give you some!

If you feel you need a material reward to reinforce some behavior, use money, books, or toys rather than anything that will confuse them about good nutrition. Still, the most successful reward I've found is the promise of *fifteen minutes alone with a parent*, whether the two of you spend that time reading, walking, or playing.

# How Much Should Your Child Be Eating?

That cute little bundle of baby fat you brought home from the hospital sure looks different now, doesn't he? Just about the time his fat wrinkles melted away last year, his food intake probably dropped as well.

Now you can catch a glimpse of his body frame as it will look throughout childhood. A lot of his appearance depends on genetics, and whether his parents are small, large, tall, or short. Much also depends on his nutritional intake and amount of exercise, especially if he plays outside or prefers to eat in front of the television.

**Food for Thought.** The TV is an often-overlooked accomplice to our faulty eating habits. After all, food companies are spending a fortune in research and production to make sure we remember their commercials. Teach your preschooler the bottom line: the companies want us to buy their products so they can make lots of money. That pretty little girl holding the candy bar is actually a well-paid actress. And that favorite athlete of ours who is hawking soda is making a lot of money to sell us something that's nutritionally inferior. Next time you're in the store with your child, look together at the labels for advertised foods: is it food to grow on? As kids grow older, they get a big kick out of making up their own commercials for their favorite foods or toys. This is one of the ways they learn about the powers of persuasion. They also become less likely to want to scarf down all the junk advertised on Saturday mornings. ■

If you feel your child is eating too much or too little, rely on your pediatrician for sound advice. By studying her growth pattern, your doctor can easily see if her caloric intake is indeed a concern.

## Failure to Gain Weight

In infants, this tendency is labelled "failure to thrive." Yet older children rarely stop eating enough to lose a serious amount of weight, according to Dr. Bart Asner.

"One of the best reasons to visit your doctor regularly is to measure your child's height and weight on a growth curve," he says. "Besides showing where an average child will be for any given age, the curve also shows if your child is deviating from the norm for his age and previous performance."

Some parents are concerned when their baby, who at first seemed to eat constantly, suddenly pushes away food and drops down toward the bottom of a growth curve. His weight reduction is usually the result of his increased activity and diminished appetite.

Our oldest daughter, for instance, was at the top of both height and weight charts when she was born, yet didn't double her birth weight until several months after her first birthday. Today, she is still slim and wiry, which tells me that this is the way her body is meant to be. No child is the same as another: if I were to line my daughter up with five friends born during the same month, they would all be of completely different weight, height, and body structure.

Growth charts, like many other medical guidelines, can be hit-and-miss affairs. Is your child relatively healthy looking, happy, alert, and active? Pay attention to these visible signs of health before worrying about where your child fits in a growth chart.

### If you think your child should be eating more:

- Space snacks and meals so that food is offered when she is hungry. Keep snacks small so they don't become meal substitutes.

- Don't serve juice at meals. Too much liquid can fill up small stomachs; instead, offer whole fruit.

- Make sure she's eating food to grow on and not empty foods that fill her with little nutrition.

And look at how the rest of the family eats. Some children want to diet like a parent, or perhaps they are intimidated by the great amount of food others quickly eat during a meal.

Some medical reasons for failure to thrive are genetics, a lack of calorie intake, or in extreme cases, severe illnesses such as intestinal or kidney diseases.

## The Overweight Child

The statistics are alarming: forty percent of all children with overweight parents grow up to be overweight adults, and at least one of every ten American youngsters is overweight.

These kids aren't aware that they're courting future heart attacks, strokes, or other serious afflictions. They only know that some of their friends laugh at them for being so inactive, and adults think they are lazy.

Although obesity may not be a concern now, your preschooler is forming habits that will dictate his future body size and health. Dr. Lendon Smith says it best: "Serve only nutritious foods. And look at what runs in your family; if your parents have diabetes, or obesity runs in the family, keep your child from becoming heavy and hooked on sweets."

**Don't harm your child by putting him on an adult reducing diet. Instead:**

- Discreetly monitor the family's habits.

- Throw out the empty calories of junk food, white flour, and sugar. Offer snacks of fresh fruit, whole milk, and other foods with essential fatty acids for their growing brain cells.

- Switch to less-fat cooking methods, such as baking and broiling instead of frying.

- Turn off the TV and go to the park more often!

- Avoid most fast-food restaurants. (See "Cold Facts About Fast-Foods" in the next chapter.)

- Give him a good example. What you serve the rest of the family is his cue as to what's good for him.

By teaching him not to overeat, you'll probably be lengthening your child's life. Laboratory studies since the turn of the century have shown that moderate eating habits can prolong life, as well as cut down on diseases.

# How Food Affects Our Brains

Your child's diet is the key to how well his brain controls his bodily functions and his behavior, including his intelligence and ability to learn. Undernutrition hinders the proper development of a child's brain, according to several experts including Dr. Carol Port.

The toxic waste from junk food was once thought to be channeled into the liver and then eliminated by our kidneys. Dr. Port believes that such waste *does* cross the "blood-brain barrier," causing cerebral allergies that can alter our minds, and even make us crazy!

"If our diets are deficient, our brains will not fire properly," she says. "There is a logical link between malnutrition and disordered brain chemistry . . . so remember that your food becomes raw material for neurotransmitters."

| Brain Fuels | Brain Impairments |
|---|---|
| Whole grain flours | Nicotine |
| Eggs, milk proteins | Alcohol |
| Liver | Marijuana |
| Soybeans, peanuts | White flour |
| Sesame seeds | White sugar |
| Other foods to grow on | Other refined, empty foods |

Of all the substances that can affect our brain, white flour and sugar are the two most common empty-calorie foods. In order to digest these foods, our body robs its own supplies of vitamins and minerals, a process which may lead to deficiencies.

Finally, sugar influences our emotional behavior by upsetting our body's level of a certain amino acid. For instance, ice cream at lunch may cause mood swings and cerebral allergies. Here is an interesting experiment which shows children the effects of what they eat. (Also see "The Kitchen As Laboratory" in this chapter for other food experiments.)

---

## Muscle Testing: A Clear Example of Sugar's Effect on the Brain

1. Ask your child to keep her arms pressed to her side, as firmly as she can, while you try to pull them away from her body to test her strength.
2. Give her a piece of chocolate. Within a few seconds, test again: her arm will weaken and float when pulled.
3. Give her a piece of apple and repeat the test. Within ten seconds, her muscles will fire strongly again.
4. Talk about how sugar/apple turns her muscles on and off. (The chocolate is immediately absorbed through mucous membranes, travels to the brain, and interferes with the firing of nerve circuits.) Eat apple for strong muscles, sugar for weak.

---

Our children's performance and behavior are also altered by exposure to toxic minerals, especially if they accumulate in their bodies. According to Dr. Port, students with elevated lead levels have been found to have greater learning problems and lower performance in schools, and possible autism. Major lead culprits include: dust, foods canned in lead (such as tuna and tomatoes), polluted air, and some ceramic glazes.

Check with your doctor if you think your child may have too much lead in her system.

# Cooking As Learning

The more you cook together, the more your child will learn about where food comes from and how to prepare it. Preschoolers marvel at kitchen miracles, such as the florets on cauliflower, or the way a raw egg becomes hard-boiled.

Next time you're making a salad together, talk about the vegetables you're putting in it and how cooking changes them. Who would ever dream that we'd get carrots and potatoes from beneath the ground? Or that tomatoes have all those seeds that squish out of their insides? (Did you know that the most nutritious part of the tomato is the jelly around the seeds?)

Try to visit a nearby farm or orchard, or read a picture book about where food comes from. Taste a just-picked apple or orange and compare it to a store-bought one. Some areas have farmers' markets where growers sell their crops, or maybe you can stop at country fruit stands while driving on your next vacation.

**Food for Thought.** Children learn to love vegetables that they've planted and watched grow. Many city kids tend balcony or rooftop gardens, or find empty lots for a neighborhood co-op garden. Horticulturist Doris M. Stone advises parents to "let the children do as much of the planting as they can, and include a few quick crops, such as leaf lettuce and radishes, since kids like instant results." For an easy indoor garden, take your child to a nursery and buy some seeds and potting soil. Next, line a few cake pans with waxed paper before putting in soil and sprinkling seeds on top. Water well, cover, and put in a closet for two or three days. Remove the cover and place the pan in a sunny window, watering every other day or so. Talk about all the changes the young plants are going through. If you're growing salad greens, harvest them with scissors and add them to a family salad. When the weather warms up, transplant the seedlings into your outdoor garden. You can get a head start on summer vegetables such as tomatoes, lettuce, and squash by starting plants in paper cups with a hole punched in the bottom. (Don't overwater, or your seeds will rot.) For a free seed catalog, write: W. Atlee Burpee Co., 19984 Burpee Building. Warminster, Pennsylvania 18974. ■

Unless your child is exposed to gardening in some way, she'll believe that food comes only from supermarkets. A friend's little girl repeatedly asked, often in tears, why her mom wasn't buying the fruit leather snacks made by the people on TV. She was afraid of hurting the feelings of the cartoon characters! Her mom immediately loaded up on ingredients for homemade fruit leather, and the two of them shared a fun morning of making their own.

Of course, we don't always have the patience and time to share a leisurely afternoon cooking or visiting farms with our children. For that five o'clock hour when you're hurriedly throwing dinner together (and your preschooler is clinging to your legs like a leech), have some back-up diversions handy. Here are some ideas that keep preschoolers entertained with a minimal need for supervision:

## For Those Times You *Don't* Want Help In The Kitchen

- Keep a stash of toys or books by the phone, ready to pull out

- Give your child some sheets to drape over a table for a castle

- Collect old buttons and macaroni in a box with yarn for stringing

- Set aside a special drawer of crayons, paper, glue, and fabric scraps for creative moments

- Give him some beans or colored macaroni to rinse, dry, and glue onto paper plates

- Hand him empty egg cartons and paper cups to stack

Even if your child isn't by your side, let him nibble while you're working. Don't we all cherish memories of licking beaters and bowls? Turn such tasting joys toward whole foods.

For example, cheese is irresistible once you've grated it, and carrots taste so much better right after you've washed them yourself. By letting him sample freely rather than forcing his ravenous tummy to wait until dinnertime, you'll keep your child better nourished and happier at the table.

If your little one rejects spicy foods, let him help you make enchiladas and sample the beans or meat while you're "building" them. He can still have a plate of fruit and cheese for dinner, and your meal will be much more enjoyable.

Such pleasant experiences build his foundation for future eating habits. In addition, cooking sharpens his reading, math, and social skills as he learns to work with other people. Your small preschooler is well on his way to making his own decisions, and wants to learn how to make the best ones.

## First Lessons About Foods

One way to interest a child in food is to relate it to something she loves. A bike-riding kid, for example, will pay more attention to whole wheat bread if she learns that she'll have more energy (and go faster) after eating it.

**Food for Thought.** Be honest when you talk about food. If you're a vegetarian because you object to animal slaughter, or if you avoid artificial colorings that are potentially cancer-causing, say so. But don't paint dramatic pictures that can terrify a youngster or turn her into a "health food snob." Personally, I shy away from telling children that any food has "poison" in it. Once they hear that some great-tasting food can kill you, they'll watch Aunt Bertha shoveling it down her throat and wonder why she doesn't fall over right there. They just might ask her. Some ideas are meant for older ears. ■

As your preschooler experiments with cooking and foods, she'll undoubtedly settle on some healthy favorites that she feels should be in every meal *forever*. Now's the time to mention how our bodies need a variety of foods so that we can have more energy, run faster, grow taller, and be happier.

As she helps you select oranges at the market, for example, say that they're good for us and help us stay well. Even a two-year-old can absorb knowledge about the four food groups, which will someday help her plan healthy meals.

## Learning Food Groups

One idea that has worked for both preschoolers and older children I've known is the presentation of the food groups as a rainbow. First, draw a rainbow with four stripes on a piece of paper.

Your child can color it, maybe even with glitter, and put it on the refrigerator for a day or so.

Next, make another rainbow picture and talk about how each stripe can be a different type of food: protein, dairy, grains, and fruit and vegetables. Label each group.

Talk about your favorite foods in each stripe, and cut out food pictures from old magazines. See which foods belong to which group, and make a collage to join the new rainbow on your refrigerator.

**By hearing casual mention of the food groups from time to time, your child will begin to check for herself what she's eating and whether she "makes a rainbow."**

When your child learns which food belongs to which color, help her plan a family breakfast and hand her a rainbow sticker to place on her wonderful menu. Older children may soon be ready to chart several meals and go shopping for ingredients. They'll enjoy seeing how many of their favorite nutritious foods can be included.

"Making rainbows" can be expanded to attain other nutritional goals. For instance, one Scout troop wanted to help the neighborhood needy by distributing food baskets, but first the girls needed a fun way to learn about nutrition in order to decide on a menu. They earned money to buy the food by doing special chores at home, and then assembled their harvests. A surprise ending was that the girls used most of their cherished rainbow stickers to decorate the food baskets!

Under the guidance of such quiet lessons, a child soon realizes that fatty, chemical-laden, processed, and sugary foods don't really have a place in his rainbow. Without being smothered in boring lectures, he's also learning a new appreciation for responsibility and family roles. ("Hey, Mom! This lunch isn't a rainbow! Can we have an apple or something from the red group?")

# Seeing Is Believing

As your child grows, she'll see for herself how different foods can affect her. My older, more emotional daughter realizes that too much junk food at birthday parties often leads to tears. Yet her younger sister, the more logical of the two, was skeptical until she tried some tests of her own, which I heartily recommend.

# The Kitchen as Laboratory: Some Great Food Experiments

1. Craving soda pop? Let your child measure out *ten teaspoons of sugar* . . . that's how much is in that 12-ounce can.
2. Read the label together. How many ingredients are unpronounceable? What are they, and are they good for our bodies?
3. Ask your dentist for some spare loose teeth. Put a tooth in each of three glasses, one filled with plain water, one with sugar water, and another with cola. Within a few days you will see the cola's acid eating through the tooth enamel. Also rotting is the tooth dunked in sugar water.

Talk about these results with your child. If sugar water and soft drinks eat away our teeth, what are they doing to the rest of our body?

Try this exploration of living things: begin by asking your preschooler how he knows something is living. (It grows and needs food.) See how a living thing absorbs food by putting celery stalks for a day or two in water with different food colorings. As your kids watch the red dye travel up the celery, mention how nutrients travel through their bloodstreams. Don't we want good food going through our bodies?

Such experiments are visual demonstrations to a child of why what he eats should be food to grow on. If he's used to good food from home, and you've taught him how to cope politely with outside offerings, he won't be as prone to peer pressure and junk food when he visits friends or eats in restaurants.

# Manners Unlimited

Every parent cringes at his child's table manners at one time or another. One father, for example, routinely despairs of his family's table etiquette just before Christmas dinner, when his relatives judge his children by whether they talk with their mouths full or put their elbows on the table.

Today, while your child still wants to imitate you, is the ideal time to talk about how to act at both Aunt Helen's Thanksgiving dinner and Bobby's birthday party. Our kids depend on us to teach them manners, especially since their future relationships can be influenced by whether they thanked their buddy's mom for a cookie, or politely asked a teacher for some extra help. Kids with bad manners are often thought of as spoiled and insensitive, while polite children are well-regarded by adults and peers. These fortunate children have modeled their manners after their parents.

Suppose your children bicker and yell at the table: call for a few minutes of total silence before explaining why it's impolite to interrupt each other. Kids throw tantrums if you inadvertently teach them that tantrums are a sure way to get attention; simply remove the offender from the table and ask him to return once he's back in control.

And make sure everything your kids need is already on the table so you won't have to jump up at their every whim. While dinnertime is a great time for conversation, it's also a time to eat. Ask your child to excuse himself when he is done eating, and take away his plate when you clean up the rest of the dishes.

## Common Courtesies

If you say "please" and "thank you" to children, they'll believe that such pleasantries are normal and natural. Even a two-year-old can politely ask to be excused from the dinner table. These good manners will result in more constructive attention and affection from others.

Of course, some behavior can't be expected at this age. If your son prefers to use a spoon rather than a fork, just smile and wait for his hand coordination to catch up to your expectations. If he constantly complains about his portions, let him spoon his own food onto his plate.

# Easy Etiquette for Preschoolers

**Passing eating utensils.** A knife, fork, or spoon should be passed by the handle so nobody gets cut or jabbed.

**Asking nicely for something**, instead of reaching across somebody or stretching across the table, is polite.

**Trying a little bit of everything** that is served. Try to ignore weird faces when your child scorns a certain food.

**Being cheerful at the dinner table** and talking about pleasant subjects makes the get-together more enjoyable.

**Learning to say "May I be excused?"** or being quiet during grace is within the range of a two-year-old.

**Cleaning up.** Preschoolers love to sponge-off a table or unload plastic glasses from a dishwasher. They can also take their own plate and cup to the kitchen sink.

**Sharing your harvest.** Teach your preschooler the joys of giving to others. Let him plan and cook a treat for a sick neighbor or special friend.

**Creating centerpieces.** While Mom or Dad is making dinner, a youngster can take charge of mealtime decorations. The next time you're buying produce ask your child to pick out some colorful items to fill a wicker basket. Or steer her toward some pretty paper napkins that will make dinner seem more like a party.

Food throwing, spitting, or other obnoxious behavior must be stopped immediately, without the offer of rewards for better behavior. Otherwise your children will expect bribes for manners that should be everyday habits.

As your child gets older, you can use dining out as an incentive for great table manners. Take her out alone and enjoy each other without making it a strained event. She'll see how other people behave, and she'll want to copy her gracious parent. Her increasingly polite behavior will let you breathe easier at Christmas dinner and all through the year.

# Eating Out: What to Expect, and What Can Drive You Crazy

Scene One. The young parents gaze in pride at their daughter as they celebrate her first birthday in a lovely French restaurant. Their darling smiles, then flings a large piece of steamed squash over her shoulder. The scorned vegetable lands on the intertwined fingers of a romantic couple who aren't thrilled. As the family makes a hasty exit, Daddy mutters, "I told you we shouldn't go to a place that doesn't have high chairs!"

Scene Two. The same family, two years later. Their oldest daughter is now a polite three-year-old who loves to eat out. It's her younger sister's first birthday, and the happy group visits the local pizza parlor. Everything goes smoothly until Mommy notices Uncle Robbie's worried face: he's scandalized that his young niece is banging her metal high chair tray with a spoon. The remaining pizza and salad is wolfed down, the birthday partiers quickly disband, and Mommy whispers to Daddy, "I told you we shouldn't go out with anybody who hasn't had kids of his own."

Scene Three. The same family, four years later, during their son's first birthday dinner at a California waterfront restaurant. The oldest daughter is scanning the menu for calamari, the five-year-old requests sushi, and Daddy is outside watching the noisy birthday boy run amuck. As Mommy sits back and enjoys the company of her daughters, she thinks, "Isn't it wonderful that we all go out to eat together!"

**Let's face it: eating out with children is not the same as before you were parents. Elegant dining is only elegant when your children are older.**

Some parents firmly believe that you should bring your children wherever you go. We agree, but only because we stopped going anywhere except family places until our children were old enough to sit through a meal, or felt comfortable with babysitters. The sooner children experience adult restaurants, the sooner they feel comfortable with new people and situations. Playhouses, restaurants, and any places with sophisticated ambience are meant for those who truly enjoy being still for over five minutes. While your three-year-old might enjoy sipping orange juice in a hotel lobby and listening to a piano player, he won't savor a leisurely seven-course dinner with the aplomb of a grown-up.

This doesn't mean that you're stuck with take-out or delivered foods if you want to take a break from cooking. Just as living with a preschooler presents unique challenges, there are ways to discover child-friendly restaurants where everybody can have a great time.

## In Search of Kid-Friendly Restaurants

Thanks to the recent baby boomlet, such places are much easier to find. They all share the same goals: the speed and efficiency to serve your meal within a few minutes after you ordered it, the informal kind of atmosphere that welcomes small, loud voices, and a gracious enough staff of people who won't comment on the pile of crumbs you have on the floor.

---

## Dining Out With A Small Child?
## Call First and Ask:

- What time is best for family dining?

- Is there a child's menu, or can you get small portions? (Often the grown-up fare is more nutritious than the greasy "kiddy-specials.") Is there a charge for an extra plate?

- Are there high chairs and booster chairs? Do you need a reservation for a booth?

- What are some of their popular whole food entrees?

- Is there a salad bar, whole grain bread, or soup that can be served quickly?

---

Ask your friends with small children which restaurants they recommend. One family we know practically lives at a Mexican place that keeps chips and salsa on the table at all times. By feeding their children some healthy snacks beforehand, they can let the little ones eat their fill of tortillas and take occasional bites from the grown-ups' plates. Everybody comes away thrilled with dinner!

Try any place with a salad bar. Children love filling their own plates when fresh fruit and raw vegetables are so attractively displayed. Even a one-year-old is captivated by a piece of watermelon and a mound of garbanzo beans, and a preschooler can be inspired to make his own salad bar at home.

One of the tricks of dining out is to know the ins-and-outs of restaurant high chairs and booster chairs. Some upscale models don't have a belt to fasten your child in, and he'll soon discover he can stand up and use the carved rails as a ladder. On the other hand, you might get an older, metal tray variety with a safety belt that seems better designed for punishment than safety. But if you don't use its belt, he will happily drum on the metal tray until he discovers how to slither out the bottom.

If you have a choice, pick a sturdy highchair with a *clean* plastic tray. You might want to bring your own portable seat that can fasten to the table (check first with the restaurant). Your child will feel at home, and you'll feel more comfortable, too.

## Planning for the Best Time

Here are some further guidelines which may make your dining experience a (happily) memorable event. The bottom line: only go to restaurants where you won't be upset when your child acts his age.

- If possible, sit in a booth (preferably by a window) so that your active child won't have to be tied down until the hot food is served.

- Try to sit somewhere without low decorative shelves and lots of knick-knacks.

- Remove other temptations before your youngster spots them: full glasses of water, knives, flower vases, abundant china coffee cups, and so on.

- No matter where you are, it helps to pull out your stash of distractions before your child gets too squirmy. Some essential car or purse tools: a cup from home, crayons for doodling on paper placemats, a small notepad, surprise toys, favorite books.

- If you bring juice or food from home, don't offer it until your food arrives. That way, your child will eat with everybody and won't be full and squirmy too soon.

- Before the waiter arrives, talk about the menu and let your child choose between a couple of items, and order himself.

- Ask for a cup with ice and your preschooler can watch it melt on saucers, pour the cubes from cup to cup, and suck on them.

- Of course, even the best-planned meal can be a disaster. Maybe your child just isn't hungry, or perhaps you need to visit a park prior to asking him to sit quietly in a restaurant. Try calling in your order ahead of time so that your food will be served right after you're seated.

- Two-year-olds are especially wary of new places, and may throw tantrums to show their fear of strange restaurants. Some cuddling and a favorite book can do wonders in such cases, as can a short walk outside. And you can always package the food to take home!

Some establishments will lead your child on a kitchen tour, which provides a unique lesson about food and how it changes. After your tour, you'll certainly know whether you want to eat there again!

As parents, we need to choose restaurants wisely, with a sense of humor and lots of patience. As your child becomes more familiar with dining out, he will develop a tantalizing taste of the adult world.

**Food for Thought.** Restaurants aren't the only places with tours for preschoolers. If you have a whole grains bakery nearby, ask to visit while the baker is making bread. (How does he bake his bread compared to your method?) For other outing ideas, check with your local librarian, Chamber of Commerce, or your state's tourist agency. Look in the phone book for food producers, such as canneries, grain mills, and egg farms. Such "field trips" make great birthday parties, too. ■

---

## FUN IN THE KITCHEN
## WITH YOUR PRESCHOOLER

*Now that your preschooler has mastered eating skills and is accustomed to all sorts of solid foods, he's probably bored with what's been served lately. Appeal to his inquisitive mind with:*

Alphabet Recipes

Blender Fruit Punch

Slow-Cooker Loaf

Grow Your Own Sprouts

Hungarian Goulash

Make Your Own Shake

Oven-Fried Chicken

---

# 6 HEADING OUT:
## Off-To-School Food

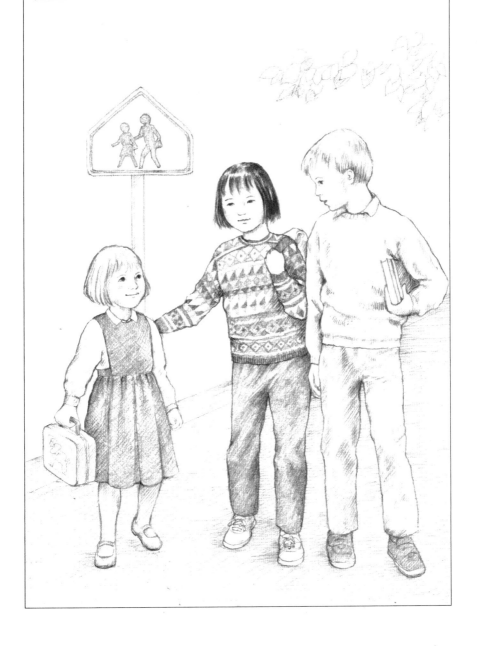

## Between Five and Seven Years of Age, Most Children

- use a knife and fork
- independently choose their friends and activities
- form their own sense of self as school expands their horizons
- make great strides toward reading, reasoning, and other mental skills
- excel in fine motor skills as well as rough play

**S**CHOOL: NEW friends, a longer academic day, and greater nutritional needs. As discussed in previous chapters, the food your child eats may help determine everything from her IQ to her coordination. It can affect her ability to listen to her teacher, to write her name, and to decide between a lunchbox or a brown bag. Such seemingly "small" decisions are forerunners of bigger choices. You should begin giving your kids the chance to choose some things without being smothered in parental preferences.

Figure out which issues aren't earth-shaking. If you don't care whether your child has a sandwich or a muffin for lunch, give him the choice. Let him decide whether soup or chili should go into his thermos. Can he choose between two outfits as you lay out his clothes for the next day?

You can spot those school kids whose parents always handle life for them. They're either frozen to a chair or frantically misbehaving in hopes of getting help from anybody, whether a teacher or a louder schoolmate. They are also the ones who will later seek out a clique of kids to dictate rules to them.

# What to Feed Your School-Age Child

Most parents don't worry about whether their school-age child is eating enough. He is perfectly capable of opening the refrigerator door and eating ten dollars worth of groceries before you even know he's home from school. With an active school-age child, your menu shifts to quick meals and snacks that can keep your child at the table long enough to relax a bit.

Your child needs food to keep up with both his weight gain and energy expenditure during the day. Especially high on his list of daily needs are proteins, fruits, and vegetables, as well as:

**Four or more servings** from the milk and cheese group, such as ½ cup milk or buttermilk, 2 cubes or slices of cheese, ½ cup cottage cheese, or ½ cup yogurt.

**Four or more servings** from the fruit and vegetable group, such as one vitamin C-rich fruit (medium orange, half grapefruit, slice of melon, ½ cup broccoli, tomatoes, etc.), ½ cup lightly cooked vitamin A vegetable (carrot, spinach, sweet potato, etc.)

**Four or more servings** from the whole grain bread and cereal group, such as: ½ cup cooked brown rice, pasta, or cereal, 1 slice of bread, etc.

**Two or more servings** of high quality protein, such as 2 medium or 1 large egg(s), 4 tablespoons natural peanut butter, 1 cup cooked dried peas or beans, 2 small slices lean meat, fish, or poultry.

My favorite way to give older kids quick access to vegetables is to keep plenty of raw carrots, celery, and broccoli available. I've found that our children will eat much more if I hand them a raw vegetable rather than a cooked one. Dips make vegetables especially enticing.

To satisfy their need for fruits and vegetables, give children a fruit at each meal, along with a potato or other vegetable during dinner. If you find your child too busy to slow down for a calm meal, make sure he finds plenty of nutritious snacks in the pantry and refrigerator.

While a preschooler may actually forget her hunger, a school-age child should not. Quietly slip her food to grow on while she's reading or doing homework. The extra nutrients will help her brain as well as her attitude!

# What To Do When Your Child Enters the Junk Food Zone

With his first taste of peer pressure, your school-age child might try to turn the family table into a real battleground. Do everything to keep from falling into this no-win contest. Loving relationships can be ruined by parents trying to control their child's selection of food (or friends). It's time to trust that your example has taken root, and to keep relationships healthy and calm on the home front. Now that he has so many new buddies, your child will undoubtedly be invited to more birthdays of the "Superhero Sugar" theme. There will be countless classroom parties with bountiful candy, red punch, and hot dogs. He must feel free to choose for himself whether to eat this food or not, without fear of parental disapproval.

There are so many more important issues to worry about than junk food! Today's child faces crucial decisions each day on the playground and in the classroom, and doesn't need parents who can't see the bigger picture. Sadly, I've known several children who apparently decided to stop confiding in their parents rather than face punishments for their less-than-ideal food preferences.

In other words, try not to overreact to relatively small pressures. A child who is used to his parents' rantings and ravings soon learns to ignore them. Don't punish a kid who makes himself sick on candy bars; instead, save your voice and energy for the time when a truly threatening temptation, such as drug abuse or drinking, rears its head. The judiciously spoken "no" is a great parental tool. By employing it as seldom as possible, a parent will be more likely to get her child to listen when he does hear it.

**Food for Thought.** Next time your child is party-bound, prepare him for the onslaught of sugar and chemicals. In my experience, it's best to keep things quiet just before the party; the sheer anticipation makes things crazy enough. About half an hour before the event, give him high-protein foods so he won't be ravenous and more likely to overeat. If your child is especially sensitive to party food, hand him some extra supplements, especially vitamins C, $B_6$, and calcium. Such precautions can make all the difference. ■

"It's certainly the parents' responsibility to try to give their kids a good diet and supportive system at home," believes Dr. Lendon Smith. "Feeling good is part of a good self-image . . . and the kid who's raised on healthy food will return to it once he realizes that he doesn't feel good otherwise."

## Be Prepared With Healthy Look-Alikes

If your child is sensitive to what others think of his food, stock up on look-alike foods that resemble what his friends eat. Bring your own canned juice or healthy sodas to the next picnic where other kids will be chugging the popular brands. Try to make your homemade fare look as "normal" as possible by perhaps leaving sprouts out of a sandwich, or buying bread that's not quite as coarse and dark as your usual loaf.

**One boy was thrilled when his mom switched from honey to pure fruit preserves for his peanut butter sandwiches. "You know what, Mom?" he excitedly told her, "Now I can squish the bread together so the jam oozes out and it looks like a normal peanut butter and jelly sandwich!"**

Keeping the junk food question small is often a question of being prepared. I know many parents who quietly keep sugar out of their home and don't make a big fuss if their kids get candy and sweets elsewhere.

One mom feeds her son a nourishing snack just before leaving for church, then doesn't overreact if he reaches for a cookie. The boy now refuses most junk food. "I can't play tennis as well once I eat it," he says. He is secure enough to refuse foods he doesn't want without drawing attention to his food preferences.

Another friend of mine keeps a stash of fruit-sweetened goodies in her purse to offer when needed. Her child has the freedom to sample poor-quality foods, yet usually prefers the more wholesome kind. Having been raised with whole foods, she doesn't crave artificial energy boosts.

Still another parent forbids her child to eat anything other than her homemade food. Her son, who has been denied junk food, has also been deprived of the chance to learn for himself. His mom now despairs at the candy wrappers she finds stuffed in his pants pockets and hidden away throughout the house. By taking his choices as a personal slur against her, she leaves herself open to feelings of guilt and manipulation. What a sad way to live when food becomes an issue rather than a joy!

- Give your child lots of healthy choices.
- Keep your home full of interesting foods to grow on.
- Don't worry if he eats an occasional doughnut!

"It scares me how many more parents are trying to run their kids' lives," says one veteran teacher. "It's as if Mom and Dad think they can keep their child from falling, or crying, or ever growing up. But that kid is just going to grow up warped, unable to find a basis for his later decisions."

# Avoiding Health Food Snobbery

It's one thing to ask Grandma not to stuff your son with chocolate chip cookies. But don't expect your child to become a pillar of strength, stalwartly denouncing all junk food. Other kids will immediately pounce on this "health freak" and do their best to break his convictions.

For instance, one little boy announces, "I can't eat this pink frosting because it has sugar!" at a birthday party. Once the others hear him, they immediately stuff M & Ms into their mouths and dare him to do the same, which he ultimately does.

**There's a fine line between teaching our kids to say no and making them worry about every scrap of food they eat. Children follow the examples they live with, so concentrate on doing your best at home!**

One of the most stressful periods of my life was when I worried about all the awful snacks our firstborn was fed at pre-school. In my fanatical devotion to food to grow on, I lost sight of the fact that she wasn't going to die from occasional lapses in her otherwise superb diet.

Now our beautiful seven-year-old knows full well the consequences of her food choices, and she makes them freely. Last Valentine's Day she ate chocolate kisses at her class party, and later told us, "Sorry about being such a grump, but I ate some candy. Think I'll go take a hot bath to calm down."

A similar example comes from pediatric nutritional consultant Sarah Bingham. "Our homes are the strongest educational grounds we have for our kids, and we can teach them with an open-handed approach. For instance, I wouldn't bring sugar into my home because it would be more expensive on my end, since my son would get sick more often. And he understands that."

**It seems that all parents wage at least one doomed battle for their kids. While I chose food as a major concern, some parents feel just as strongly about certain playmates, designer clothing, or other issues that kids decide for themselves, anyway.**

We should simply do the best we can at home, and try to relax in public. Just as you discipline your child with love, you can tenderly teach him how to eat well. A simple "Sorry, we don't eat that" can sometimes satisfy a request, as can some nonlecturing words about our need for good food so we can play, think, and look our best.

**Food for Thought.** One of the most heartbreaking food reactions in older kids is bed-wetting, which may be the result of allergies. A study by the American College of Allergists determined that cow's milk caused bed wetting in sixty percent of 500 children studied. Eggs, grain, and citrus were other common allergens. If your school-age child is still bed-wetting, let him know that you love him by helping him solve the problem, or by showing him that something positive is being done. It's not his fault, and shouldn't cause the tension, guilt, and embarrassment he may feel. Take the opportunity to learn more about how food plays a part in his physical and mental health, and how allergies often show up in strange ways. ■

There's a lot you can do to make your home teachings stay with him at school. Pack enticing lunches that leave other kids green with envy for whole foods. (See "Lug-Along Lunches" at the back of this book.) You can also begin a groundswell battle for better nutrition in the schools, which is what some parents have already successfully done.

## Joining the Volunteer Ranks

As far as I'm concerned, those adults who volunteer their time and energy to help in the classroom, Scouts, or other kid groups are quiet heroes. As a nutrition-minded parent, think about joining their ranks. You'll add some say-so to the type of foods that are served. Classroom parent-volunteers, for example, can either make party goodies or call others and ask them to contribute specific items. I've found that the parents are usually the ones to insist that junk food must abound at every gathering.

At one Brownie meeting (as leader, I had asked parents to bring only nutritious snacks), one mom actually apologized to the girls for serving sliced oranges instead of candy or cookies! Yet the girls didn't seem to feel they were being short-changed.

---

## Snacks That Win With Kids of All Ages
### (Often, it's all in the packaging!)

- Cubes of different cheeses, or wafers shaved off with a cheese plane (served with a bit of apple for palate-cleansing)

- Bagels and cream cheese (optional: add caviar)

- Stuff-your-own celery with cream cheese or peanut butter

- Anything made on the spot, such as peanut butter balls (and other recipes at the end of this book)

---

Snack time can become an adventure with just a little imagination. At one Daisy Girl Scout meeting, a creative mom brought each girl a small straw basket, then showed them all how to place lettuce leaves and raw vegetables around the sides. After adding a small cup of dip in the center, each girl was thrilled to eat from her own attractive vegetable basket!

Look at the calendar and choose a theme when you volunteer to feed your children's friends. Fill a piñata with peanuts, coins, and toys, or fill plastic Easter eggs with stickers and pennies. Kids love any snack if you wrap it in rainbow cellophane.

**You'll soon have your own crazy stories about teachers, P.T.A. leaders, and others who can't imagine kids being happy without doughnut holes and chocolate milk. But junk food doesn't *have* to be the center of attention at every social gathering.**

Just laugh off all the good-natured ribbing you'll get for being a "health nut," and quietly plan the next camp breakfast or school fundraising dinner. Think of yourself as a sneaky champion of kids' rights, while other grownups thrill to see you doing the work.

There are some instances in which silence doesn't get the job done. Room parents can have a lot of control over the type of foods served in the classroom, but they usually have no voice whatsoever as to what those students are served in the school lunchroom. But it doesn't have to be that way.

# Battling the School Cafeteria

Do you ever get a chance to see school food? In the interest of lower costs and kids' preference for "fast-food," many districts serve the likes of bright pink hot dogs, greasy hamburgers, and fried fish sticks. These delectables are usually served with white bread, pickles, French fries, and a pudding popsicle or imitation ice cream cup.

Pizza is another cafeteria workhorse (bleached white flour crust with enough preservatives to make it last a year, fake cheese, weird sauce), often offered twice a week because it satisfies the grain, dairy, and vegetable requirements of a state-approved nutritious lunch. As a dismal encore, students are served chocolate milk or fruit punch. Or they can help themselves to even worse food from vending machines.

## Poor School Food Leads to Poor Performance

Pity the children whose growing bodies daily absorb all the fat, chemicals, and salt in these meals. And think twice about letting your child eat food prepared by nutrition "experts" who regard catsup as a vegetable.

Even the most wholesome breakfast may not prevent your child from having an awful afternoon once his body has to cope with such junk. Yet if you ask why more fruit and vegetables can't be added to the menu, as I once did, you may hear a cafeteria worker sniff, "Don't be silly, we served green beans a couple times and the kids threw them away. You don't want them going hungry, do you?"

Let's hope that sort of thinking is slowly changing, due in part to modern crusaders who are de-junking school menus. By learning how to grow and prepare their own nonprocessed foods, children are also learning why their bodies respond so much better to their needs.

**Food for Thought.** It's a fact. Kids greatly improve their school performance after sucrose and food additives are reduced in their school lunches. A recent four-year study of over 800 New York City schools showed that dietary changes caused test scores to jump from eleven points below the national average to five points above. Eliminated or reduced were: two synthetic food colorings, sucrose, synthetic flavorings, and additives BHT and BHA (both are allergens and suspected carcinogens). ■

What a tremendous gift to give kids: the ability to do so much better in school by simply eating a wholesome lunch.


## Nutra: A Program for Intelligent Eating

Food to grow on is just one part of the Nutra program, a brainchild of Sara Sloan while she was head of the food and nutrition department of Fulton County's school system (Atlanta, Georgia). Sloan's motto of "Eat to Learn! Learn to Eat!" could stand to be posted on the refrigerator doors of parents everywhere as they teach their children more about food choices.

Nutra kids quickly learn to appreciate good food by cooking in their classrooms and sampling future cafeteria meals. Instead of lunching on processed junk, Nutra students "intelligently eat" such meals as sesame chicken with wheat germ gravy, tossed green salad with cottage cheese dressing, cracked wheat bread, fresh fruit, and milk.

**This good food is boosting the kids' academic scores as well as giving them energy, sunny dispositions, and a willingness to learn. It's no wonder that the Nutra program is being requested for classrooms from Illinois to Indonesia.**

"These nutritional ideas are not for everyone, only for those who wish to feel better," says Sloan. By convincing kids that whole foods are fun to prepare, tasty, and good for them, the Nutra program provides incentives for entire families to eat well.

Why buy the "Superhero Sugar" stuff that makes kids dopey in school and impossible at home? With a little instruction, school-age children can see for themselves how much better they can feel.

How about you doing some of the teaching yourself? Big kids are just as crazy about cooking for themselves as preschoolers are, and will gladly wolf down the healthy food they despised before they learned how to prepare it. Think about donating a slow-cooker or toaster-oven to your child's classroom, then volunteer to teach cooking!

## Creative Classroom Cooking

- Demonstrate the marvels of sprouting.
- Dry fruits and herbs for other recipes.
- Fix a class lunch, such as pita tuna sandwiches.
- Make English muffin pizzas.
- Put together a potluck salad bar.

Divide the class into smaller groups, with one grating cheese, another preparing sauce, and a third boiling noodles for a spaghetti party. For one cooking class, I had everybody knead a quick bread. Then, while the bread was baking, one group shook cream into butter, another mashed strawberries for jam, and a third made fruit salad.

**Some kids have never seen or tasted a cake made from scratch. It's a real joy for them to assemble wholesome ingredients rather than just add water to**

**a boxed cake mix. They'll see various ingredients (eggs, flour, milk, butter) miraculously transform into a very different product. And it's a great lesson in label reading.**

Once kids realize the difference, they'll probably go home and scour their own pantry for boxes to label-read. This kind of lesson is especially valuable when you take your kids shopping and they clamor for the most popular brown-bag items.

**When an older child reads that those "natural" granola bars are actually stuffed with sugar, chemical marshmallows, and fake chocolate, his desire for them will diminish. Same for those packages of peanut butter and "cheese" crackers; although they're cute in their cellophane with their little plastic knives, the ingredients are usually far from wholesome.**

Instead of throwing money after unhealthy snacks, spend a little more on some fun picnic supplies and make your own, or shop around a bit. Most health food stores have a wide selection of fruit leather, granola bars, and cookies that are fruit-juice sweetened, yet packaged to look just like the popular junk advertised during Saturday morning cartoons.

## BEANS: Another Heroic Group

One more Pied Piper for food-to-grow-on-kids is Anastasia Condas, founder of BEANS (Better Educational and Nutritional Standards), a special interest group of the California Reading Association. While BEANS is a hands-on program carried out in local schools, it also works on the state and national levels to raise the nutritional consciousness of parents and educators.

BEANS offers creative suggestions for you to improve the school cafeteria. Begin by finding out if your school's P.T.A. has a nutrition committee and if not, start one. The National P.T.A. has guidelines that tell how twenty state P.T.A.s improved school nutrition programs. Also write a blurb for the school newsletter, or ask around for other parents interested in improving cafeteria food.

Next, evaluate your school's classroom situation. See if there is any nutrition instruction, especially within the health or science curriculums. Write to your state capital to learn what training programs are available for classroom use. Your child's teacher is already overworked, and will be grateful for any materials you can offer.

Finally, find out if teachers can work with cafeteria staff on projects. Might students be introduced to new foods with taste-testing parties?

"Be prepared to go to the top," advises Condas. "Talk to the principal, the district head of food service, the superintendent, and the board. When I lodged my campaign against junk food, I found a kindred spirit in the president of the Board of Education!"

**You'll gain even more support if you're well armed with information. BEANS, Nutra, and the Center for Science in the Public Interest are just a few of the sources that want to help.**

The key to your success is to remain polite and keep a sense of humor, so that you won't be brushed off as a parent obsessed with yet another flaky program. With help from other parents, you can call for a Board of Education policy on junk food and nutrition.

"We had wonderful cooperation from the local papers and a local doctor who was interested in environmental illnesses," says Condas. "Basically, we told the schools to practice what they preach." Considering what's at stake, yours will be a grassroots campaign worth winning.

**Food for Thought.** Even if your child brings her own lunch to school, or if your school doesn't have a cafeteria program, find out about lunchroom policies. Is food sharing allowed? (If so, pack extra goodies for your child to give away so she won't be as likely to trade her food for Twinkies from another kid.) What is the social climate in the cafeteria? In one exclusive private school, parents pay nearly five dollars a day for their kids to eat hot lunches prepared by a master chef. Yet sometimes the food supply runs low, and a few students end up with only mashed potatoes. One mom decided to start sending lunch to school with her daughter, only to discover that brown-baggers had to sit in their own corner apart from those purchasing lunch. Find out if any elitist policies are at work in your own school. Kids have the right to a wholesome and pleasant meal.

■

If you're a room parent, you may be able to start your own hot lunch program. Scout-out the prices of some health food sandwich shops and make up a list of three choices. If your school has cooking facilities, help the kids bake a big pan of lasagna, or show them how to broil their own natural burgers to go on whole wheat buns. Use the time to bring out the differences between their sandwiches and the kind available at fast-food restaurants.

# Cold Facts About Fast Foods

Hold onto your hats. And your stomach. Of all the research on nutrition, the latest data on fast-food is among the most disturbing. Kids should definitely know about it, and so should their parents, who spend nearly fifty billion dollars a year on the stuff.

Even if you never drive through those golden arches, your child will probably be handed a fast-food burger at some after-soccer lunch. Or somebody will bring a platter of fried chicken nuggets to a neighborhood get-together. One well-meaning room parent I know often spends nearly twenty dollars on milkshakes to "treat" the class during a hot day.

Maybe the soccer coach isn't aware that he's handing his players more salt than they should consume in an entire day. And the neighbors probably don't realize they're also eating fatty chicken skin and MSG. Or maybe they do know, but aren't informed enough to care. Those ravenous kids certainly won't read the ingredient list for their frosty chocolate shakes:

| | | |
|---|---|---|
| milk | corn sweetener | partially delactosed nonfat milk |
| sugar | cellulose gum | mono- and diglycerides |
| water | guar gum | karaya gum |
| cream | sodium citrate | cocoa processed with alkali |
| whey | carrageenan | dipotassium phosphate |
| salt | sodium carbonate | sodium phosphate |

And perhaps: caramel color, artificial flavors, potassium sorbate, Blue Dye Number 1, Red Dye Number 3, and sodium alginate.

Do you ever go to the store to buy a box of potassium sorbate and a quart of Red Dye Number 3? Do you put them into the food you cook at home? Why accept them in fast (or any other) food?

According to Michael Jacobson, executive director of the Center for Science in the Public Interest and author of *The Fast-Food Guide: What's Good, What's Bad, and How To Tell the Difference,* we should steer our families away from the worst offerings from fast-food land. Not only will our lifespans be lengthened, but our wallets won't feel the hefty sting of paying so dearly.

"We have to remember that most of us cannot afford the calories that come from eating fast-foods on a regular basis," says Dr. Judith Anderson, a nutrition professor and dietician at Michigan State University. "In fact, routinely eating fast food can be a real problem for children's nutrition."

## Choosing Wisely in Fast-Food Land

Anderson and others regard the brightly colored "kiddie packages" offered at most major chains as one of the most expensive and cholesterol-loaded choices available. They usually consist of a greasy hamburger, sugary soft drink, oozy french fries, and a token toy. Kids would fare better at fast-food places if their parents ordered milk and fresh fruit for them in place of the fatty alternatives, or if the kids ordered these things themselves.

"Actually, the first thing parents should do is turn off the TV set," urges Jacobson. "Kids are really brainwashed into thinking a hamburger, french fries, and cola is where it's at. We should be choosing roast chicken and other low-fat alternatives, such as broiled fish, potatoes (but watch out for all those stuffings), and salads."

You can avoid a lot of chemicals and calories by removing the skin from fried chicken and scraping off the condiments. For those who desire red meat, a roast beef sandwich is a lot lower in fat than a hamburger.

"You know, a five-year-old who eats fast-food isn't going to develop fat-related disease within the next year," notes Jacobson, "but he is forming his eating habits that will last a lifetime. Even if your child isn't in dire danger of a heart attack, he should get used to eating good food."

**To avoid temptation parents can bring along their own food, or rely on supermarkets for convenience. Many markets now feature delis, spruced-up produce sections, and ready-to-eat food departments.**

With a little sleuthing, you may uncover some local health-minded restaurant managers. Some franchise owners are disregarding corporate policy and using vegetable oil rather than beef fat or coconut oil for their fried foods.

## Some Truly Independent Franchisees

Ken Raffle, co-owner of four Arby's Restaurants in Maine, caters to a large crowd of folks who love tabouli, brown rice, and a house salad dressing of vinegar, oil, and lemon juice. "People who come to us say they don't eat in other fast-food restaurants because they have to sacrifice their normal eating patterns," he says. Besides offering whole wheat hamburger buns and local crab and lobster, Raffle features apple cider as an alternative to soft drinks. His salad bars, made up of locally grown organic vegetables, sell two to three times more than the average fast-food restaurants.

Another independent soul with a heart of gold is Carolyn Duncan, owner of C. J. Carryl's in Muncie, Indiana. Faced with her own high blood pressure, high blood cholesterol and triglycerides, Duncan set out to devise a non-greasy way of cooking chicken. Her method of "hot-air popping" transforms chicken, catfish, and other commonly fried foods into healthy alternatives with great flavor. C. J. Carryl's also offers freshly steamed vegetables, a sulfite-free salad bar, and mashed potatoes with gravy.

"Just like you have to watch what your kids see on TV, you also have to watch what type of fast foods you feed them," Duncan believes. "Make sure those foods are low-fat and low-salt, and really check it out when somebody says their stuff is nutritious."

One final example of the "fast-food can be health-food" principle comes from Paul Wenner, owner of Wholesome and Hearty Foods in Portland, Oregon. His meatless Gardenburger is taking the West Coast by storm, with astronomical sales to airlines and grocery stores that want to offer a meatless burger. Each patty is made up of fresh mushrooms, fresh onions, rolled oats, low-fat mozzarella and other natural cheeses, brown rice, egg, bulgur wheat, walnuts, and natural seasonings and spices. It has no added salt, one-fifth the fat of a regular hamburger, and only half the calories. In addition, it comes frozen and can be heated in your toaster. Who says we can't have fast-food convenience at home?

**Food for Thought.** The success of these restaurateurs proves that we, the buying public, can be responsible for what the big chains offer us to eat. For better or worse, fast-food is now part of our national identity; tens of millions of Americans eat it every day. And we're suffering the consequences of heeding those billion-dollar ad campaigns: per capita, our soft drink consumption has more than tripled since 1951, sugar intake has increased 40%, and we eat about 14 pounds of French fries each year. Yet even the huge conglomerates are sensitive to consumer pressure. More of them are offering sulfite-free salad bars, beans, and non-fried, healthier meat dishes Their changing menus are clear examples of public pressure at work. If enough of us ask for fast-food to grow on, the system will respond. ■

As parents concerned about our children, we need to know what they're eating. Perhaps there should be laws requiring package labelling on the scores of fast-food dishes available. We can read a label before we give our child something from the supermarket, so why not when we buy a pre-packaged hamburger?

Even better, how about making fast food at home? Next time you make bread, freeze some extra dough for a quick pizza crust. Or keep some pre-formed patties and whole grain buns on hand for your own burgers. Besides avoiding the commonplace chemicals and saturated fats of the restaurants, you'll discover your own specialties.

It's a good time for the great taste of *your* cooking!

# Making Sure It's Safe

Okay, our families are thriving on their diets of fresh produce and whole grains. Like millions of other Americans, they're eating less meat and junk food. Surely we're on the right track to better health.

Yet if only those foods could talk, we'd hear some pretty interesting stories of how they came to be . . .

Consider the apple we tuck in our kid's lunchbox. It's shiny and gorgeous because it's been sprayed with pesticides an average of fifteen times, treated with chemical washes in the packing house, and then waxed to a high gloss.

That apple may be permeated with captan, parathion, and daminozide. Carrot sticks can hold trifluralin, chlorothalonil, and linuron. A bunch of grapes is often riddled with methyl bromide, and potatoes may be treated with aldicarb. Even the milk served at school can be harboring aflatoxin, clorsulon, fenbendazole, and thiabendazole. And all of these chemicals are known or suspected carcinogens!

Without a doubt, our food supply is contaminated with invisible pesticides, drugs, preservatives, and germs. According to Americans for Safe Food, a new consumer coalition, we need to know about such dangers. As we shall see, with a bit of extra effort they can be avoided.

**Food for Thought.** The watchdog of our nation's food supply, the U.S. Food and Drug Administration, is also warning us that food-borne bacteria is at a crisis level. According to FDA Commissioner Frank E. Young, his agency cannot always adequately monitor our food safety because of budgetary constraints. In fact, two new problem areas—imported foods and meals consumed away from home—have alarming levels of pesticides, bacteria, and other various harmful chemicals. And we're paying for such contaminants: food-related illnesses may be costing us one billion dollars each year in medical bills and absences from work.

The F.D.A.s advice? Says Young, "Consumers need to read, be informed, and protect themselves." ■

Some of our elected representatives believe that our government isn't moving fast enough to get rid of all the substances tainting our food. Congressman Ted Weiss (D-N.Y.), chairman of the House Subcommittee on Intergovernmental Relations and Human Resources, says that it's up to us to clamor for the right to know the dangers of the foods we're eating. "Government regulators have been allowing contaminants to remain in our food supply for years after they have been identified and their risks disclosed," Weiss says. "In light of the persistent refusal of government agencies to protect the public from thousands of potentially dangerous chemicals in our food, mobilizing consumer demand for safer food is essential."

The committee has reported on countless food safety problems, including unsafe food color additives, pesticides in food, and residues of the drugs given to animals. Our meat, milk, and egg supplies are especially impure.

**Pesticides are also invaders of our food chain. And over eighty percent of these farm chemicals have not been tested to determine whether they are cancer-causing.**

Weiss and others praise "Americans for Safe Food" as an example of important consumer steps to demand foods free of dangerous additives. "I am hopeful that one result of a successful campaign will be consumers who, armed with greater knowledge about chemical and bacterial adulteration of their food, will demand accountability from industry and Government agencies charged with safeguarding the public health," Weiss says.

So where do we start?

## The Campaign is Underway

Whether you work within a national campaign or not, there is a lot you can do as a family to push for safe food. Petitions are now circulating which urge Congress and the President to develop and enforce laws to make contaminant-free food available to all Americans. (As one friend told me, "I'm not sure I would ever choose to give up all my sulfited-shrimp and dyed cookies. But I sure should have the right to know what I'm eating!")

Once we know the realities, we can look for safe alternatives. Local coalitions can meet with consumer affairs directors of local supermarkets, urging them to offer contaminant-free food. These markets can also be asked to label the colorings, drugs, waxes, and pesticides used in or on fresh foods, or to post signs and provide pamphlets with this information. Local directories of markets, farmers, health food stores, and co-ops that offer safer food can be prepared.

In response to such consumer demand, some trailblazers are now offering food free of dangerous contaminants. H. J. Heinz makes its baby foods solely from produce that has not been treated with any of twelve pesticides labeled potentially hazardous by the Environmental Protection Agency. And the 125 outlets of Safeway's United Kingdom division offer organically grown fruits and vegetables. Wouldn't it be nice for American consumers to receive the same pure food?

## A Lifetime of Good Eating

With these changing attitudes in mind, you'll find it easier to feed your family well. When you give your kids food to grow on, you're giving them a better future. You're also helping them along the road to choosing a lifetime of good eating.

Here are some quick, easy, and delicious recipes to start you toward that end.

---

### FUN IN THE KITCHEN WITH YOUR SCHOOL-AGE CHILD

Cooking can be as good as homework for developing your child's reading, addition, and motor skills. If she is a little rusty at math, bring her into the kitchen and ask her to measure some ingredients. She'll enjoy cooking even more if you quietly supply her with ways to feed her friends. Our daughters have friends who ask to come over for a tea party, which is nothing more than dressing up in play clothes and eating cream cheese and jelly sandwiches that are trimmed with cookie cutters. The key is to let kids make their feast by themselves, including serving the treats on a pretty platter in another room.

*Other recipes for school-age chefs:*

Breakfast Apple Cobbler
Charna's Creamy Carob
  Candy
Dressed-Up Burgers
Fluffy Eggs

Make Your Own Salad Bar
Nachos With A Flourish
Whole Wheat Pancakes
  or Waffles
Whole Wheat Pizza

---

# RECIPES

# Recipes for Food to Grow On

**N**OBODY LIKES all foods. But there are some tried-and-true recipes that hit the mark most every time, and these are the ones I've included to make mealtimes happier and healthier. All of these dishes have been made, or at least helped along, by children who have judged them tasty enough to share with others.

Many of the recipes include questions which may help you talk about the food with your helpers. Preschoolers, for instance, are inherently curious and love to see how yeast makes bread rise, or how cheese makes a sauce thicken. Once they realize that everyday cooking is an ongoing science experiment, their perspective changes forever, and so does their interest in what they eat.

There are many natural foods cookbooks at your library and bookstore which can help your family enjoy food to grow on. Use them. I've found that mealtimes become pretty hurried and silent when our menus sink into a familiar rut. With just a little encouragement, children can help make a dish that's really special. So cook with a child at your elbow and a smile on your face.

Hey kids! Here are some ways to get cooking:

- Before you cook, make sure there's somebody older around (like a parent) to help you get started. Read the recipe first to see if you have everything you need.

- Get everything out ahead of time. Here are some of the common tools you'll need: measuring cups and spoons, stirring spoon, cookie sheet, frying pan, rolling pin, grater, electric mixer or hand beater, pot or pan, griddle, pot holder, and masher.

- Follow the recipe carefully and ask for help.

- Clean up, and you'll be welcomed back to cook again!

# 7 FIRST FOODS

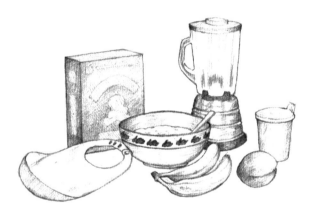

# Equipment for Your
# Natural Baby-Food Kitchen

- Washable highchair (try to get a tray with a lip) or clamp-on baby seat

- Small eating utensils such as demitasse spoon or dishwasher-safe plastic baby fork and spoon

- Plastic or other unbreakable bowl and small plate with lip

- Bibs—not the cute small ones, but the jumbo, wipe-off variety, or diapers and small dishtowels

- Apron for you, if you're spoonfeeding

- Old shower curtain or sheet to go under highchair

- Plastic baby cup with detachable top

- Paring knives to chop foods, skin apples, and so on

- Vegetable scrubbing brush for washing produce

- Vegetable steamer to fit inside saucepan

- Small saucepans for heating tiny portions

- Blender to puree chunky family foods or whirl drinks (Be careful not to overblend—it just takes a few seconds!)

- Spatula to scrape sides of blender

- Food processor to grate cheese, slice small pieces of meat, and do much of the blender's work

- Baby food grinder, an extra-handy, portable tool for purees

- Storage containers for extras, with covers
(But don't save any uneaten food from baby's dish, since saliva from feeding spoons causes bacterial growth in leftovers.)

# First Foods for Six-Month-Olds

For optimal nutrition, lightly cook foods from the following list, or leave them raw. For spoonfeeding, puree in a blender or a baby-food grinder, or mash with a fork. Don't give baby any leftover pulp or seeds. For finger-feeding, either grate food or finely chop it. Some fruits and vegetables may be served raw. An older baby will enjoy chunky-textured food, such as lumpy oatmeal. These are also some of the least allergenic foods.

**Yellow vegetables.** Squash makes a great first food.

**Whole grain rice, oats, or barley.** Mash or serve as cereal without cow's milk or sweetener. Add other grains after you know your baby suffers no allergic reactions.

**Banana.** A nutrition-packed, portable food.

**Applesauce.** Unsweetened and uncooked. Simply whirl some apple slices in your blender.

**Papaya.** Babies love the bright color.

**Chicken.** Well-cooked and finely chopped.

**Breadcrusts.** Whole grain and toasted. Great for teething and chomping, toast can be enjoyed with a "jam" puree of a favorite fruit or vegetable.

# Terrific Teething Foods

The poor darling! Some babies have teeth that pop up unnoticed, yet yours is suffering from throbbing gums before the first speck of white enamel is visible. He might find comfort in nursing; afterwards, hand him a natural teether to chew on. Not only is he developing muscle coordination, but he's getting a taste for food to grow on!

**Breadcrusts.** Well toasted, whole grain. You can save "heels" in the refrigerator; chilled crusts are often rock-hard and nicely cold on baby's bare gums.

**Bones.** A special favorite is a chicken leg bone, which is just the right size for a teething baby to chomp on and wave around. Once your baby is used to bits of chicken, hand him a bone without the cartilage, skin, and most of the meat. Some families who love ribs also fix one without sauce and eat off most of the meat, then give their baby the bone to teethe on.

**Carrot.** Make sure it's a nice fat one. Carrot sticks are too small and a teething baby might break them into small, chokeable pieces. Clean, chilled carrots are lovely. If teething is especially trying, stick a carrot in the freezer for a while.

**Celery.** Some babies love to chew on a stalk of celery, but for some reason our kids seemed to know just how to gag on any strings they gummed away from the stalk. Try it with caution.

# Second Stage Foods:
# for Older Babies with Teeth

After baby tries and enjoys the above foods, she can branch out and include family favorites. Just continue to introduce one food at a time, with patience. By placing one food at a time on the highchair tray or plate, you'll also be reducing the chance for spectacular messes. (But expect them, just the same!) Now for some new tastes:

**Beef.** Extra lean, finely chopped.
**Various poultry.** Skinned, well-cooked, and finely chopped.
**Pasta.** Or other form of any grain already introduced.
**Egg white.** Use whole egg very sparingly before first birthday.
**Pears.** Best fully ripened and raw.
**Avocado.** Raw and peeled.
**Peanut butter.** Creamy, natural unsweetened, unsalted.
**Potatoes.** Sweet and white.
**Broccoli**
**Peas**
**Cauliflower**
**Dried peas and beans.** Sparingly in case of gas.
**Spinach.** Eat immediately after it's been prepared.
**Corn**
**Green beans**

**Cantaloupe and other melons.** Great as slush when whirled with a bit of banana.
**Mangos**

And try combinations, such as apple-banana, applesauce-squash, mango-pear, carrot-squash, etc. Mixed flavors can help introduce a new food, or reawaken baby's taste for an old favorite. Carrots and peanut butter make a nice spread, and spinach pureed in a blender makes a tasty spaghetti topping. Other great mashed partners include sweet potato-avocado, carrot-white potato, and any combination of the above-listed foods you can think of.

# Third-Stage Foods: for Babies Nine Months and Older

Now, for babies who are nearly ready for family casseroles:

**Tomatoes, pureed.** Dip fresh tomatoes in hot water for ease in peeling, then whirl in a blender and strain to remove the seeds. Makes a good juice that can also be mixed with whole grain pasta.
**Cottage cheese**
**Natural cheese.** Uncolored, non-processed.
**Yogurt.** Use unflavored, unsweetened yogurt, or you can add your own unsweetened fruit.
**Whole egg, scrambled.** Add it to cereal and fruit puree.

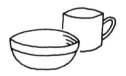

# Don't Feed Your Baby These Foods

*Some of these sweet, salty, refined foods can actually harm your child's growth; many are likely allergens, and others can cause choking in a small child. Try to eliminate any refined, empty-calorie foods from your kitchen. Your child's tiny stomach and growing brain need the most nutritious, pure food to grow on you can give her.*

AVOID ANYTHING artificially colored, sugar-sweetened, salted, or adulterated with additives. The only sweetener, if any, should be fruit juice.

BACON
CANDY
CAKES AND CRACKERS*
CANNED FOODS
CARBONATED DRINKS
CHEESE, IF PROCESSED
CHERRIES, IF COLORED
CHIPS, INCLUDING Cheese Puffs, Corn, Potato
CHOCOLATE
CITRUS FRUITS AND JUICES
COCONUT OIL
COFFEE
CONDIMENTS, INCLUDING horseradish, catsup, hot sauce
COOKIES*
CROISSANTS
DESSERTS*
DIABETIC FOODS*
DOUGHNUTS
EGG WHITE
FATTY FOODS
FLAVORED GELATINS
GRAPES
HAM
HONEY (FOR CHILD UNDER ONE)
HOT DOGS

ICE CREAM
INSTANT FOODS
JAM, JELLY*
MARGARINE
MEATS, IF PROCESSED, INCLUDING bologna, pastrami, salami, other luncheon meats
NUTS
PASTRY
PICKLES AND PICKLED FOODS
PIE*
PREPARED DELI FOODS, INCLUDING coleslaw, chicken salad, pasta salad, sauerkraut
RYE BREAD
SALAD DRESSINGS
SALT
SAUCES
SAUSAGES
SHERBET
SMOKED FOODS
SOFT DRINKS AND SODAS
SUGARS AND OTHER SWEETENERS, INCLUDING Aspartame, brown sugar, corn syrup, fructose, honey, molasses, maple and other syrups
WHITE BREAD

* Only use whole grain, unsweetened, and unprocessed foods.

# Kitchen Rules and Tools

- Nurse your baby before feedings.

- Serve home-prepared, whole foods.

- Relax and make meals pleasant.

- No solid foods until around six months or older.

- Start with one food, a teaspoon at a time, for three days or so. Watch for allergies before adding other foods.

- Hold off on sweets, salt, condiments, hard-to-chew foods. Also delay commonly allergenic foods.

- General rule for pureeing or simmering: one tablespoon of water or breastmilk per piece of *fresh* fruit or vegetable.

- General rule for freezing: double the above and fill the individual slots of an ice cube tray. Cover and freeze. About an hour before feeding baby, remove one cube and let it thaw to room temperature. Try to use it soon. Don't refreeze any food, and throw away leftovers.

- Best cooking methods: steaming, broiling, or baking. Avoid canned and commercially frozen food, if possible; at the very least, rinse off any salt or sweet syrup.

- Vegetables and fruits: wash everything first and peel to remove any trace of pesticides from the skin. Start with lightly steamed yellow squash and other vegetables before adding the sweeter taste of fruits such as banana. Mash for spoonfeeding, or finely chop for finger-feeding.

- Whole grains. Start with soft-cooked rice, oatmeal, or barley and moisten with breastmilk or water. Offer toasted bread crusts, mashed grains, or cereals.

- Meats. Skin all poultry before cooking. Grind or chop well-cooked chicken. Babies love to gnaw on a chicken bone, minus the cartilage, skin, and most of the meat.

- Other high-protein foods. Beans, peas, lentils, peanut and other nut butters.

- Juices. Use sparingly; rely instead on whole fruit for extra vitamins and fiber.

- Eggs. For the older baby. Start with egg yolk, given whole or mashed, moistened, and spread on a bit of bread. Some babies love a bit of scrambled or soft-boiled egg; hold off on anything fried.

- Dairy products. For the older baby. Delay cow's milk until after twelve months. Non-allergic babies often love yogurt and natural cheeses.

- Combining foods. After two foods have been tried singly, you can mix them together. A year-old baby can eat anything from spaghetti to chop suey, if he's not sensitive.

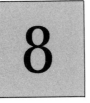

# 8 BREAKFASTS
## *Alternatives to the*
## *Boxed Cereal Rut*

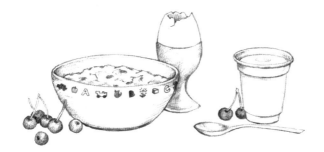

# 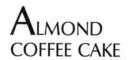LMOND
## COFFEE CAKE

PREPARATION: 20 MINUTES
COOKING: 6 MINUTES
YIELD: 6 SERVINGS

*Commercial coffee cakes are usually colored with a yellow dye to seem egg-rich.*

**2 cups whole wheat pastry flour**
**2 teaspoons baking powder**
**¾ cup light honey**
**1 egg, beaten**
**1 cup plain yogurt**
**1 teaspoon pure almond extract**
**½ teaspoon grated lemon rind or lemon juice**
**½ cup raisins**
**½ cup almonds, chopped**
**¼ cup finely grated coconut, unsweetened**

**Topping:**
**¼ cup milk**
**¼ cup butter**
**¾ cup almonds, chopped**
**½ cup light honey**

CAKE: Preheat the oven to 350°. Sift together flour and the baking powder and set aside. In a separate bowl cream the honey and then add it to the flour. Mix the egg, yogurt, almond extract, and lemon and add them to the flour mixture. Stir in the remaining ingredients and pour into an 11-inch by 13-inch pan.

TOPPING: Bring the milk, butter, and almonds to a boil. Add honey and pour over the cake. Bake for 30 minutes.

# Breakfast
## APPLE COBBLER

PREPARATION: 10 MINUTES
COOKING: 3–9 HOURS
YIELD: 4 SERVINGS

*Compare the tastes of different types of apples with your child. Which color and flavor are favorites?*

**4 medium-size, tart apples**
**¼ cup honey (optional)**
**1 teaspoon cinnamon**
**¼ cup melted butter**
**2 cups natural granola-type cereal, with fruit and nuts, or add
    your own raisins**

Core and slice the apples, then place them in a slow cooker and mix in the remaining ingredients. Cover and cook on low for seven to nine hours, or on high for two to three hours. If you fix this before going to bed, you'll smell breakfast when you wake up. Top with milk for breakfast; left-overs make a great dessert with ice cream or whipped cream.

# Cottage
## CHEESE-YOGURT
## PANCAKES

PREPARATION: 5 MINUTES
COOKING: A FEW MINUTES
    PER BATCH
YIELD: 6 LARGE PANCAKES

**½ cup cottage cheese**
**½ cup plain or fruit yogurt**
**3 eggs, beaten**
**½ cup whole wheat flour**
**1 teaspoon pure vanilla extract**

Mix all the ingredients by hand or with a beater until well blended. Fry on a hot, greased griddle until steaming and golden on both sides. Serve with honey or fresh fruit. Fresh berries are terrific!

# Delicious Mush

*This food was a real staple of colonial times, when Pilgrims called it "samp."*

*Stoneground cornmeal is milled from the whole grain and tastes wonderful. It's a pale color as opposed to the weird bright yellow we usually see.*

**6 cups cold water**
**1½ cups stoneground cornmeal**

Bring four cups of the water to a boil over medium heat. Mix the cornmeal with the remaining two cups of cold water until smooth. Add this to the boiling water and stir until thick, about two minutes. Then turn down the heat and simmer, stirring often, until the mush is as thick as you like it, another two minutes or so. Spoonfed babies like it a bit runnier than you may prefer, so scoop out a bit while it's cooking and let it cool for baby. Older kids love to watch the bubbles come to the top of the mush and break apart. Spoon into bowls.

**FOR OLDER TASTES:** Serve with milk and perhaps a dollop of molasses or honey. Any leftovers can be pressed into a greased loaf pan and chilled. The next morning, dip slices into wheat germ and fry in a bit of butter. Eat like pancakes.

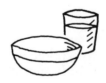

# Easiest-Ever Granola

PREPARATION: 15 MINUTES
BAKING: 60 MINUTES
YIELD: ABOUT 6 CUPS

**3 cups rolled oats**
**1 cup raw wheat germ or wheat bran**
**½ cup sesame seeds or shelled sunflower seeds**
**1 teaspoon cinnamon**
**½ cup cooking oil**
**½ cup honey or molasses**
**2 teaspoons pure vanilla extract**
**1 cup nuts, chopped**
**1 cup dried fruit, such as raisins or chopped dates**

Preheat the oven to 275°. Combine the oats, wheat germ, seeds, and cinnamon. Mix the oil, honey, and vanilla and pour over the oat mixture. Stir to coat evenly and spread in a large baking pan. Bake for 60 minutes, stirring every 15 minutes. Break up large lumps and add the fruit and nuts. Refrigerate.

# Fluffy Eggs

PREPARATION: 5 MINUTES
BAKING: 5 MINUTES
YIELD: 2 SERVINGS

*A favorite recipe for preschoolers to cook with you.*
*Fertile eggs have more food value than the supermarket variety, and are usually fresher.*

**2 eggs     2 slices whole grain toast, buttered**

Preheat the oven to 350°. Gently crack open an egg and separate the yolk from the white, leaving the yolk in the eggshell and putting the white in a bowl. Repeat with the other egg. Use an electric or hand beater to beat the whites until they are stiff enough to form peaks. Put half the fluffy whites in a mound on each piece of toast. Then use a spoon to make a little hollow in the center of each mound. Gently slip one egg yolk into each hollow. Bake on a cookie sheet until the whites are brown and the yolks firm, about five minutes.

# GRAHAM'S OATMEAL PLUS

PREPARATION: 2 MINUTES
COOKING: 5–10 MINUTES
YIELD: 4 OR MORE
SERVINGS

*Eggs make this oatmeal a complete protein.*

**2 cups oatmeal, not the "instant" variety**
**2 tablespoons wheat germ (optional)**
**4 cups milk**
**½ cup or more raisins**
**2 eggs, beaten**
**Toppings: cinnamon, butter, honey, sliced bananas**

Mix the oatmeal and wheat germ and set aside. Measure the milk into a saucepan and add the raisins. Heat until boiling. Add the oatmeal, stirring for a minute or two, then turn down the heat. Cook for a few minutes and stir to test whether enough water has been absorbed. Just before the mixture thickens, stir in the eggs and cook a bit longer. Arrange toppings on table and serve the oatmeal in bowls.

**LEFTOVER OATMEAL LOAF:** Pour leftover cooked cereal into a greased bread pan. Refrigerate until the next morning, then turn out and slice. Dip slices in cornmeal or wheat germ, and fry in a bit of butter or oil. When crisp, top with applesauce, cinnamon, or other pancake toppings.

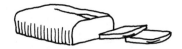

# Make your own corn flakes

PREPARATION: 10 MINUTES
BAKING: 1 HOUR
YIELD: 1 CUP

¾ cup cornmeal, whole grain yellow
⅓ cup cold water
⅓ cup thawed apple juice concentrate

Preheat the oven to 250°. Mix everything in a bowl and pour over an oiled baking sheet. Bake for one hour, or until crisp. Crumble mixture with your fingers and then store it in an airtight jar.

# Surprise apple pancakes

PREPARATION: 10 MINUTES
COOKING: A FEW MINUTES
    PER BATCH
YIELD: 4 OR MORE
    SERVINGS

2 cups whole wheat flour (or 1½ cups flour and ½ cup wheat germ)
1 tablespoon cinnamon
2 teaspoons allspice
1 teaspoon nutmeg
2 teaspoons baking soda
1 banana and one apple, sliced
2 eggs, beaten
2 tablespoons oil or melted butter
2 tablespoons honey or molasses (optional)
2 cups buttermilk

Mix the flour, spices, and baking soda. Add the fruit and stir gently until blended. In a separate bowl, mix the egg, oil, honey, and buttermilk. Add the dry ingredients and stir just until blended. Fry on greased griddle at low temperature so the fruit won't burn. Great topped with yogurt and fruit, or yogurt and jam. Leftovers can be frozen and later warmed up in your toaster.

# Whole Wheat Pancakes or Waffles

PREPARATION: 5 MINUTES
COOKING: A FEW MINUTES
PER BATCH
YIELD: 4 SERVINGS

**4 cups buttermilk or yogurt or sour milk**
**4 eggs, beaten**
**½ cup oil or melted butter**
**4 cups whole wheat flour (1 cup cornmeal, wheat germ, oats, or other grain may be substituted for 1 cup of flour)**
**4 teaspoons baking soda**
**2 teaspoons cinnamon**

Beat together the buttermilk, eggs, and oil. Mix in the dry ingredients. You can also add one cup of thinly sliced fruit or berries. For waffles, pour part of the batter in the waffle maker, sprinkle with fruit or nuts, then cover with more batter. For pancakes, pour the batter directly onto a hot greased griddle. Cook until they stop steaming and are nicely browned.

WHAT'S YOUR FAVORITE PANCAKE TOPPING? Before you choose maple syrup, read the label to make sure it's real. Also delicious are applesauce, cream or ricotta cheese, peanut butter, warm butter and honey, yogurt, fresh fruit or preserves, and so on.

# 9 LUNCHES
*Lug-Alongs, Salads,
Spreads, and Favorite
Noontime Finger Foods*

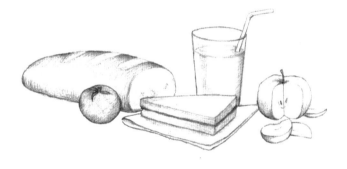

# Luscious Lug-Along Lunches

After a morning of play or school, kids need a sturdy lunch to keep them going strong. Try to give them the most appealing, favorite foods, including:

- two protein choices, such as crackers and cheese or celery sticks with peanut butter

- at least one fresh, raw fruit or vegetable

- a nutritious sweet treat

- a healthy drink (but not too much lest they fill up on juice)

- and another tempting food

As one who has packed lunches for years, I can safely say that there are three major challenges to brown-bagging for kids—keeping foods the right temperature, making whole foods look "popular" and respectable (let your child make his own lunch as much as possible), and avoiding the sandwich burn-out. I've found that packaging can solve many such quandaries.

The best way I've found to make lunch special for a school-age child is to include a note. For years I've tucked a small note in lunches, especially if our children wondered what I did while they were in school. Before they could read, for example, I'd draw a picture of me working at the computer, or perhaps sketch a picture of the beach if we were heading there after school.

Or simply draw an eyeball, heart, and "U" in a line for "I Love You." As your child grows, you can write in cursive handwriting, which kids delight in deciphering. One mom hollowed out an apple and tucked a note inside. A little flag on a toothpick stuck in the apple said, "Look inside for a surprise! I'm sure proud of you!"

Corny, huh? Sometimes, on especially harried mornings, those notes are the last thing on my mind. But they've become an expected part of our daily routine. Even my children's classmates look forward to the notes I send.

# Luxuries for the Well-Dressed Lunchbox:

**Unbreakable Thermos.** A small, narrow-mouth one for hot and cold liquids; a wide-mouthed thermos for soups, yogurt, other spoonable goodies.

**Paper bags.** Avoid thin brown bags, which often tear and leak. Decorate insulated bags with rubber stamps and stickers.

**Unusual lunchboxes.** Use straw mini-baskets or personalized boxes.

**"Show-Off" tools.** Send along an apple corer and slicer for your older child, who will also eat several hard-boiled eggs if he can use an egg slicer himself.

**Special touches.** Party cups, plastic utensils, paper doilies to use as a "tablecloth".

Try to do anything you can think of to make lunch special for your student. She's gone through a long, hard morning and can use a little encouragement from the loving homefront. Notes, stickers, toys, favorite foods, all are reminders that you love her and care enough to do a little extra. Even on those PB & J days.

## Sandwiches: the New, the Old, the Novel

Sandwiches can be a real bore and a nutritional disaster for those kids who constantly face bologna, mayonnaise, and white bread. To make your wholesome sandwiches exciting:

- Choose different loaves, such as bagels, pita, muffins. Be sure you're buying wholegrain. Some "whole wheat bread" is actually white fluff with caramel coloring.
- Soggy sandwiches? Send plain bread, and pack spreads in cups so your child can make his own repast.

- Freezing sandwiches? Butter both slices to the crust before spreading on wet fillings.

- Sandwich boycott? Try muffins, small fruit juice-sweetened pies, and other wholegrain goodies. Your child's favorite homemade cookie may be just as nutritious as two slices of bread.

## Favorite Sandwich Spreads

- The infamous peanut butter and jelly, made with natural peanut butter and unsweetened preserves. Variations: other nut butters, cream cheese, or kefir cheese. Great with bananas, apples, dates, raisins, sunflower or sesame seeds, or unsweetened applesauce. For nut butters with more nutritional punch, blend in some milk powder or wheat germ. Or fold in some grated lemon rind or tomato juice.

- Tuna, usually made with a dab of mayonnaise or sour cream. Add chopped tomatoes, relish, a dash of mustard, or salsa for zing.

- Sliced white cheddar or Jack cheese sandwich. Especially good with sliced tomatoes and sprouts if your child likes them. Try cheese, sprouts, and sliced apple, too.

- Ricotta cheese sandwiches. Blend equal parts of peanut butter, soft blue cheese, or mashed garbanzo beans with ricotta.

- Cream cheese sandwiches. Good on raisin bread for "sweet" days, spread with chopped walnuts and dates. Or use bagels.

- Chicken liver pate, only if your child likes it. Mash sauteed chicken livers with hard boiled egg and a bit of parsley and mayonnaise. Or simply add a bit of sauteed onion before chilling.

- Colorful grated sandwich fillings. Mix together grated carrot, orange, and apple with peanut butter, sour cream, or mayo.

- Hard-boiled egg or chicken sandwiches. Add some grated cheese, chopped celery, chopped walnuts, and onions with a dab of mayonnaise.

- Leftover beans sandwiches. Mash cold garbanzo or pinto beans, and add chopped nuts, guacamole, or avocado slices with lemon juice, sliced tomato, and lettuce.

- Roll-up sandwiches. Use spinach or lettuce leaves instead of bread around a creamy filling. Or use a rolling pin to flatten bread before adding spread. Secure with toothpicks. Our daughters love to roll up a stick of cheese in a slice of natural bologna and fasten it with a toothpick.

# Foods for Cold Weather: Beating the Winter Chill

- If you have a small insulated thermos, pack favorite soups, stews, hot carob and other drinks, chili, spaghetti, sloppy joe fillings, any appealing leftovers. Our kids love cups of grated cheese and sour cream to add to their lunchtime chili. Their favorite soup garnishes are crackers, grated parmesan cheese and homemade croutons.

- Some sandwiches are great if warmed just before school and wrapped securely in double heavy-duty foil. Grilled cheese, leftover pizza, fish burgers, burritos, and quesadillas can fit into insulated containers. Put a slice of meatloaf between two slices of bread, cover with cheese, wrap in foil, and bake at 350° for 15 minutes. Wrap again in foil before putting it in the lunchbox.

- Baked apples and other hot treats. Core large apple and cut in half. Place halves flat side up on individual foil sheets and stuff them with raisins, chopped walnuts, a pinch of salt, lemon juice, and honey. Wrap them tightly in foil and bake for 30 minutes at 350°. Wrap again in foil.

# Salads and Other Hot-Weather Fare: Beating the Dog Days

- A good, small thermos and insulated bags can equip a lunchbox for soups, salads, and more, such as cold dinner leftovers (especially spaghetti) and fresh fruit or vegetable salads, with dressings packed separately.

- Favorite mix-ups: cottage cheese and cold brown rice mixed with cooked peas, carrots, or raisins. Yogurt is great sent in a thermal container with a cup of granola or nuts to stir in.

- Exotic delicacies: cold artichoke hearts sent with a cup of mayonnaise and mustard, or spinach salad with oranges and grapes.

- The simplest icy treat is frozen fruit (unsweetened berries are great) packed in a pre-chilled container. The fruit will be cold and moist by lunchtime, and can even be spread on a peanut butter sandwich.

- Special treats: cold tapioca, puddings of rice or bread, raisins, fruit soups. For instance, puree watermelon, honeydew, or cantaloupe with a dash of lemon juice, and whirl with a cup of apple juice. Chill or freeze for a cool lunch.

- Put frozen boxes of pure juice (wrapped in a sandwich bag to prevent leaking) in a lunchbox to keep other foods cool.

# BREADCRUST ZUCCHINI QUICHE

PREPARATION: 10 MINUTES
BAKING: 30 MINUTES
YIELD: 6 SERVINGS

*Sauteed zucchini blossoms are a real delicacy.*

**3 slices whole wheat bread**
**½ pound sliced zucchini**
**1 tablespoon butter**
**½ pound tomatoes, chopped**
**1 teaspoon oregano**
**2 tablespoons whole wheat flour**
**1 cup cottage cheese**
**2 eggs, beaten**
**¾ cup plain yogurt or sour cream**
**⅓ cup parmesan cheese, grated**

Preheat the oven to 375°. Cut the bread in half diagonally and layer it around the edge of a 9-inch pie plate. Saute the zucchini in butter until tender; add the tomatoes and oregano and bring to a boil. Let boil, uncovered, for three minutes. Stir in the flour and spoon the mixture into the bread-lined pie plate. In a separate bowl, mix the cottage cheese, eggs, sour cream, and half the grated cheese. Spoon this over the vegetables and sprinkle everything with the remaining cheese. Bake for 30 minutes or until it's firm in the center.

# CURRY SALAD

PREPARATION: 15 MINUTES
CHILL: 1 HOUR
YIELD: 4 SERVINGS

½ cup plain yogurt
1 tablespoon mayonnaise
¼ teaspoon grated orange peel
⅛ teaspoon curry powder
1 orange, peeled and diced
2 cups cooked chicken, diced
½ cup sliced celery
½ cup coconut, unsweetened
½ cup slivered almonds

Blend the yogurt, mayonnaise, orange peel and curry powder, then chill. Put this mxture in a large bowl and add the other ingredients. Chill for one hour before serving.


# GREEN PEA SALAD

PREPARATION: 10 MINUTES
CHILL: 1 HOUR
YIELD: 4 SERVINGS

*Children love to shell peas and make sculptures or "atoms" by poking toothpicks into them. You can string them together for mobiles that will last indefinitely.*

1 pound peas, fresh, shelled
4 tablespoons grated natural cheese
4 tablespoons chopped pickles or onion
4 tablespoons plain yogurt or mayonnaise
Optional: 1 baked potato, diced

Mix all the ingredients together in a large bowl. Chill for one hour before serving.

# Grow Your Own Sprouts

*What are sprouts? Seeds, grains, or beans that are just starting to grow. After sprouting in three days, soybeans have 500 percent more vitamins.*

**½ cup seeds (mung and lentil are great)**
**Sprouting jars or wide-mouthed glass jars covered with fine screening and secured with rubber bands**

Divide the seeds between the two jars and add a cup of water. Pour off the water (this cleans the seeds) and then cover with fresh water to soak overnight in a dark, warm spot. The next morning, drain and rinse again.

Keep up this cycle at least two times a day, making sure to thoroughly drain the seeds. The more you rinse them, the faster they'll grow. In about three days, your seeds will be sprouted and ready to eat plain or added to a sandwich, salad, or omelette.

Not only are sprouts fun and easy to grow, but they guarantee you fresh, unsprayed vegetables all year round. Other types of beans or seeds to try include alfalfa, radish, wheat berries, garbanzo, soy, fenugreek, and unhulled sesame or sunflower. This is a great introduction to gardening for the young child, who will see changes every day.

Sprouting makes a great classroom experiment. Donate the supplies to your child's class and help the kids get started. Then bring in salad dressing, plates, and forks to eat the harvest.

# JOURNEYCAKES

PREPARATION: 10 MINUTES
COOKING: 2–5 MINUTES
YIELD: 2 OR MORE
SERVINGS

*Another relic of our pioneer times, when settlers would carry a big corn cake to eat during their journey.*

*This food is ideal for older babies, nine months or so, who love to hold big, round foods.*

**2 cups plain yogurt or buttermilk**
**½ cup wheat germ or whole wheat flour**
**2 large eggs**
**1 teaspoon baking soda**
**1 cup stoneground cornmeal**

Mix together all the ingredients in the order listed. When the batter is smooth, fry it like pancakes with a bit of butter to keep it from sticking. Babies love to tear these cakes apart, while older family members like to top them with fruit, yogurt, or whatever their favorite toppings are.

# MAKE YOUR OWN NUT BUTTERS

*How many nuts are in each shell? Nuts are actually seeds of the plant.*

**1 pound raw shelled nuts (peanuts are most common, but cashews, almonds, and macademias are good)**

Preheat the oven to 325°. Roast the nuts in a large flat pan, one layer deep for about ten minutes. Stir and taste them often to be sure they're roasting evenly and not burning. Then pour a small amount into a food processor or blender. Without scraping butter away from the blades, add more nuts, pushing them down. Remove after you have about a cup of butter. This method keeps you from adding more oil and ending up with greasy nut butter.

# Make-your-own Salad Bar

*Kids love to help make a salad bar for the rest of the family, and they usually eat more vegetables this way as well! While a toddler can help put celery bits into a bowl, a preschooler can wash and tear lettuce as an older sibling grates cheese or slices mushrooms. It's fun to talk about the foods while everybody is preparing them. Break open a celery stalk and feel the water inside. Mention that while the celery grew in the ground, its stem carried food and minerals from the roots up to the leaves. The sun helps make food for plants, too. We eat vegetables from all different places on a plant. Carrots and potatoes are roots, peas are seeds, and cauliflower is . . . a flower!*

## Bowls or platters of many of these festive salad makings:

Apples, chopped
Beans (garbanzo, pinto, kidney)
Black olives, sliced
Broccoli bits
Carrots, grated
Cauliflower bits
Celery, chopped
Cheese, natural, grated or cut
   in wedges
Chicken strips
Chives, chopped
Cucumbers, sliced
Eggs, hard-boiled, chopped
Green leaves, such as lettuces
   (romaine, red, butter) and
   spinach

Green peppers, chopped
   or sliced
Mushrooms, sliced
Parsley, chopped
Peas, fresh or frozen
Radishes, sliced
Raisins
Sprouts
Squash, sliced
Tomatoes, sliced
Tuna, flaked
Walnuts, chopped
PLUS: dressings, lemon
   wedges

Combine these ingredients at the table. Everybody gets a unique salad.

# Potato Pancakes

PREPARATION: 15 MINUTES
COOKING: 2–5 MINUTES
YIELD: 2 OR MORE
SERVINGS

*Older children like to look at whole potatoes before you grate them. Not only do they grow in the ground, but new plants come from the eyes of the potato.*

**3 eggs**
**1½ cups grated potatoes**
**½ cup grated carrot**
**2 tablespoons wheat germ or whole wheat flour**

Mix the eggs, potatoes, and carrots together, then stir in the wheat germ. Pat them into 3-inch pancakes and brown in a bit of butter until crisp. Babies loves the texture and the different colors.

**FOR OLDER TASTES,** serve the pancakes with applesauce. You can also add onion, or replace the carrot with zucchini.

# Pumpkin Butter

PREPARATION: 20 MINUTES
COOKING: 15–20 MINUTES
YIELD: 2½ CUPS

*This is wonderful when spread on freshly baked bread or muffins. One of our daughters prefers hers in a dish with a spoon.*

**1 can pumpkin: 16 ounces**
**½ cup honey**
**¼ cup molasses**
**1 tablespoon lemon juice**
**¾ teaspoon cinnamon**

Combine all the ingredients in a saucepan and bring to a boil, stirring frequently. Reduce the heat and simmer until thickened, stirring often (about 15 minutes). Cool, then chill for at least one hour, or freeze.

# Raid-the-Refrigerator Quiche

PREPARATION: 20 MINUTES
BAKING: 30 MINUTES
YIELD: 6 SERVINGS

*Quiches are best served lukewarm, although some kids love a piece of cold quiche for lunch.*

*If your child turns up her nose, tell her this is "cheese pie," and use Jack or cheddar cheese rather than the stronger-tasting Swiss.*

**9-inch pie shell or whole wheat pie crust**
**1½ cups milk**
**3 eggs, beaten**
**½ teaspoon nutmeg**
**1½ cups natural Swiss or Jack cheese, grated**
**3 cups vegetables, sauteed and sliced (onions, mushrooms,**
  **broccoli, tomatoes, squash)**

Preheat the oven to 375°. Heat the milk to near boiling, then let it cool a bit before adding the eggs, spices and cheese. Place the vegetables on the bottom of the pie crust and pour the milk mixture over all. Bake for 30 minutes or until firm in the center.

# Super Sandwich Spread

PREPARATION: 10 MINUTES
YIELD: 1¼ CUPS

*Plan on longer if kids are fixing their own sandwiches.*

**¼ cup honey or light molasses**
**½ cup natural peanut butter**
**½ cup wheat germ**

Blend the honey and peanut butter until smooth. Gradually add the wheat germ and stir until well blended. Spread over whole grain bread. Optional: top the spread with raisins and/or sliced bananas. It's also good when topped with a cheese slice and melted under the broiler. Cover and refrigerate any leftovers.

# Vegetable Pancakes

PREPARATION: 15 MINUTES
BAKING: 25 MINUTES
YIELD: 2 OR MORE
SERVINGS

1 large zucchini
1 large carrot
2 sprigs fresh parsley (optional)
1 cup grated natural cheese
2 eggs, beaten

Preheat the oven to 350°. Cut the zucchini and carrot into large chunks, then grind them in the blender with the parsley. Add the cheese and egg, then shape into patties and bake on a greased cookie sheet for 25 minutes or until firm.

# Zucchini Cakes

PREPARATION: 15 MINUTES
COOKING: 2–5 MINUTES
YIELD: 4 SERVINGS

*A tasty whole meal for finger-feeding babies and others.*

3 eggs
2 zucchini, grated, about ½ cup
½ cup whole wheat flour or stoneground cornmeal

Stir the eggs into the grated zucchini, then mix in the flour until all the lumps are gone. Fry the batter like pancakes with a bit of butter to keep it from sticking. Delicious topped with grated cheese.

# 10 APPETIZERS AND SNACKS

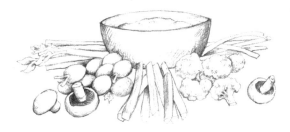

# CHEESE COOKIES

PREPARATION: 5 MINUTES
BAKING: 2–3 MINUTES

*What makes these cookies rise and fall? The fat in the cheese first melts, then runs out. Sit in front of the oven and watch!*

**Your favorite natural cheese, such as cheddar**

Preheat the oven to 350°. Cut slices of cheese into small squares about ½ inch thick. Grease a cookie sheet and arrange the cheese squares with at least 2 inches of space all around. Bake for about two to three minutes, until the edges look nicely browned and the cookies are flat.


# CHEESE AND SALSA DIP

PREPARATION: 5 MINUTES

**1 can natural salsa: 12 ounces**
**1 pound grated cheddar cheese**
**For cold dip: 1 carton sour cream: 16 ounces**

HOT DIP: melt cheese in salsa and serve immediately, or keep warm in a slow cooker. Also great on nachos.

COLD DIP: combine the ingredients and then chill for about an hour. Delicious with crackers and raw vegetables.


# CHUNKY ARTICHOKE CASSEROLE

PREPARATION: 10 MINUTES
BAKING: 15 MINUTES
YIELD: 4–8 SERVINGS

*Serve as a dip or over pasta.*

**4 small jars artichoke hearts, drained, rinsed**
**1 cup parmesan cheese, grated**
**½ pound mozzarella cheese, grated**

1 cup mayonnaise
2 cloves garlic, minced

Preheat oven to 350°. Chop the artichokes and mix them with the remaining ingredients. Spread into an 8-inch by 11-inch baking dish and bake for fifteen minutes. Serves eight as an appetizer and four as a main dish.

# CRABBY MOUSSE

PREPARATION: 20 MINUTES
COOKING: 20 MINUTES
CHILL: 4 HOURS
YIELD: 6 SERVINGS

2 tablespoons unflavored gelatin
¼ cup cold water
6 ounces cream cheese
1 can cream of mushroom soup

1 cup mayonnaise
1 cup celery, finely chopped
1 small onion, grated
6 ounces flaked crab meat

Put the gelatin in the water and stir until it dissolves. Add the cream cheese, soup, and mayonnaise. Cook this mixture in a small pan over low heat, stirring until smooth. Remove the pan from the heat and add the celery, onion, and crab. Pour into a bowl or mold and chill until firm, about four hours. Invert over a serving plate and serve.

# FRUIT-CHEESE KABOBS

PREPARATION: 5 MINUTES

Shish kabob *means "sword meat."*

**Your favorite natural cheese, cut in cubes**
**Colorful in-season fruits, cut in cubes**

Poke a toothpick or skewer through the foods for a portable meal.

# Guacamole

*Stick some toothpicks into the avocado's large seed and balance it in a cup of water. Roots grow fast!*

**2 slightly soft avocados**
**2 teaspoons lemon juice (keeps the guacamole from blackening)**
**2 tomatoes, chopped**
**4 tablespoons chopped onion**
**1 teaspoon cilantro, chopped (optional)**

Mash the avocados and mix in the remaining ingredients. Serve as a garnish for Mexican dishes or as a dip with tortilla chips. You can substitute salsa instead of the tomato/onion/cilantro mixture, but try to drain off part of the water first. Serves four if you use it as a dip with chips and raw vegetables.

# Salsa

**2 large tomatoes, chopped**
**2 onions, chopped**
**1 can of green chile peppers, chopped: 8 ounces**

Stir the ingredients together, and use a food processor or blender if you like a salsa that's less chunky. Chill in refrigerator until you're ready to use it on eggs, enchiladas, burgers, and other dishes. Ideal as a topping, or melt cheese into it for a hot dip.

# 11 HOT DISHES

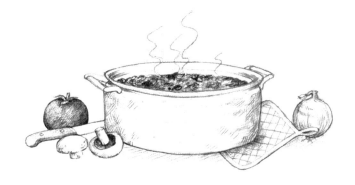

# Barbecue Anything!

*Use chicken wings, drumsticks, beef ribs, any high-quality meat with bones for handles.*

**Your choice of meat**
**Natural barbecue sauce, or use the following recipe**

BAKING METHOD: Place the meat in a baking dish and bake for one hour at 350°. If you use chicken, baste it with the sauce and return it to the oven for 10 more minutes. If beef or pork, turn the meat and drain the fat before basting with sauce. Bake another 30 minutes or more.

SLOW-COOKER METHOD: Put the whole chicken or meat pieces in the pot, pour on about 2 cups of sauce, and cook on low for 8 to 10 hours. You an also add cut-up raw potatoes, onions, and carrots.

# Barbecue Sauce

PREPARATION: 10 MINUTES
COOKING: ABOUT 20
    MINUTES
YIELD: 3½ CUPS

*Also good on scrambled eggs and burritos.*

**4 tablespoons cider vinegar**
**4 tablespoons Worcestershire or tamari soy sauce**
**2 teaspoons chili powder**
**2 teaspoons paprika**
**1½ cups water**
**1½ cups catsup**

Mix all the ingredients in a small saucepan and heat over medium heat until the tastes are blended. If you're cooking for a toddler, add very small amounts of spices. Let cool, cover and refrigerate.

# Barbecued Corn-on-the-Cob

PREPARATION: 5 MIINUTES
COOKING: 10 MINUTES

*The word "corn" often refers to a country's main crop. In England, corn means wheat; in Scotland it means oats.*

**1 ear of corn per child, husked and silked**
**butter**
**Supplies: preheated charcoal fire with glowing coals, wet newspaper or cheesecloth, foil, tongs**

Wrap clean ears in wet newspaper or cheesecloth, then cover in foil, shiny side out. Put in fire and cook about 10 minutes, turning frequently with tongs. Remove from heat, unwrap, butter and eat. This also works well as a winter treat with frozen corn.

# Bean Filling for Enchiladas, Burritos, Tostadas

PREPARATION: 10 MINUTES
YIELD: ENOUGH FOR A
DOZEN SMALL SERVINGS

**1 cup cooked pinto beans**
**2 tablespoons chopped onion**
**1 cup grated cheddar cheese**
**2 tablespoons chopped sunflower seeds or nuts**
**Optional: ¼ cup wheat germ or sliced olives**

Mash the beans and mix in the other ingredients. For tostadas, spread on tortillas and top with lettuce, tomatoes, or other toppings. For burritos, spread the beans on tortillas, roll them up, wrap in foil, and warm in a slow oven for about 15 minutes. For enchiladas, put two tablespoons of filling and one tablespoon of grated cheese on each tortilla, roll up, and place in a greased baking dish. Cover with salsa or sauce and grated cheese, then bake for 20 minutes at 350°. Serve tostadas, burritos, or enchiladas with toppings such as guacamole, chopped olives, and sour cream.

# BEANED-OUT CASEROLE

PREPARATION: 15 MINUTES
COOKING: 65 MINUTES
YIELD: 6 SERVINGS

*Ideal way to use up left-over beans.*

**6 cups tomato juice**
**1 cup cooked barley**
**2 cups cooked legumes, or combination such as: ½ cup lentils**
    **and 1½ cups pinto beans**
**1½ cups diced potatoes**
**1 medium onion, chopped**
**Pinch of thyme and parsley**

Heat the tomato juice to boiling, add the barley and cooked beans and simmer for 25 minutes. Add the potatoes, onions, and spices, simmer 40 minutes more. This dish is especially good with fresh bread or rolls.


# CHEESY MACARONI

PREPARATION: 15 MINUTES
BAKING: 30 MINUTES
YIELD: 4 OR MORE
        SERVINGS

*A combination of cheeses gives this some zip.*

**½ pound whole wheat macaroni, cooked and drained**
**2 cups milk**
**1 pound natural cheddar cheese, grated**
**¼ teaspoon paprika**
**1 cup Parmesan cheese, grated**
**2 tablespoons butter**
**½ cup crushed crakers or wheat bran**

Preheat the oven to 350°. Heat the milk. Add the cheddar cheese, stirring until it melts. Add the paprika and pour the sauce over the macaroni in a greased 2-quart baking dish. Top with Parmesan, dot with butter and crumbs. Bake for 30 minutes or until browned and bubbly.

# COMPANY CASSEROLE FOR A CROWD

PREPARATION: 30 MINUTES
BAKING: 30 MINUTES
YIELD: 10 OR MORE SERVINGS

*Freeze an extra pan for those days you just can't cook.*

**2 pounds whole wheat noodles, cooked and drained**
**3 pounds ground turkey or beef**
**1 large onion, chopped**
**½ teaspoon chili powder**
**¼ cup butter or cooking oil**
**4¾ cups tomato soup**
**3 cups corn**
**1 cup water**
**1 pound grated natural cheese**

Brown the meat and onions with chili powder in butter. Add the soup, corn, water, and noodles. Pour into a 13-inch by 9-inch pan and top with cheese. Bake for 30 minutes at 400°. Serves ten or more.

# DINNER LICKETY-SPLIT

PREPARATION: 15 MINUTES
COOKING: ABOUT 20 MINUTES
YIELD: 4 SERVINGS

*Whenever you use flour to thicken a sauce, simmer it for at least 15 minutes to get rid of the "floury" taste.*

**1-pound ground turkey or beef**
**1 small onion, chopped**
**2 tablespoons whole wheat flour**
**½–1 cup milk**

**Optional: ½ cup grated cheese, chopped vegetables**

Brown the meat and onions in a skillet. Sprinkle the flour over the meat and pour in the milk. Stir until thick, add options, and serve over toast or steamed brown rice.

# Gooey Chicken

PREPARATION: 15 MINUTES
BAKING: 1½ HOURS
YIELD: 4 SERVINGS

*How is cheese made? Rennet, which is the lining of a calf's stomach, is added to milk so that it curdles. Part of the milk turns to solid chunks called curds, and the rest is a liquid called whey. The whey is drained and the curds are salted, molded, and ripened into cheese. What did Little Miss Muffet eat?*

**3-pound chicken, cut up**
**½ cup whole wheat flour**
**½ cup cooking oil**
**1 small onion, chopped**
**3 cups chopped tomatoes**
**1 cup water**
**¼ pound natural cheese, grated**

Preheat the oven to 325°. Coat the chicken with flour and brown in the oil. Put in a baking dish and cover with the remaining ingredients. Bake for 1½ hours. Top with cheese the last half hour of baking.

# Hungarian Goulash

PREPARATION: 20 MINUTES
COOKING: 45–60 MINUTES
YIELD: 4 SERVINGS

*In the old days, folks didn't measure anything in their recipes. They just threw in whatever they liked.*
*How do we measure things now? Which is bigger, a teaspoon or a tablespoon?*

**Onions, sliced**
**Dab of oil**
**Stewing beef**
**Potatoes, cut up**
**Carrots, cut up**
**Paprika**

Heat the onions in the oil in a large pot until they turn yellow. Meanwhile, place the meat, potatoes, and carrots in a bowl of clear water. After the onion is yellow, cover it with paprika and add the meat to the pan. Do not squeeze water from meat. Let the meat simmer and brown, then add the potatoes and carrots. Simmer until the vegetables are tender. Peas or other vegetables may be added ten or fifteen minutes before serving. Great over steamed brown rice or whole wheat noodles.

# MAKE-YOUR-OWN BURGER (OR TOSTADA) PARTY

*Whether you're warming up a lentil burger or one of pure beef, add some extra sizzle with a choice of toppings. Try having a "burger-bar" party; each guest gets a plate with a whole wheat bun and patty, then chooses among garnishes such as:*

**Cheese slices (cheddar, Swiss, Jack, etc.)**
**Onion slices**
**Tomato slices**
**Lettuce or spinach leaves**
**Salsa**
**Refried beans**

**Sour cream**
**Sauteed mushrooms**
**Peanut butter and jelly**
**Avocado bits or guacamole**
**Chopped hard-boiled egg**
**Jalapeño peppers**
**(and whatever else sounds good)**

The above suggestions also work great for a **tostada party.** Everybody takes a whole wheat tortilla (chapati) and layers it with their favorite toppings. You can also set out plates of shredded chicken and other salad fixings.

Or **make-your-own burrito:** spread refried beans and grated cheeses on a tortilla, roll it up, wrap it in foil, and warm it in the oven. Great with a dollop of sour cream, salsa, and chopped onions.

# MIGHTY MARINADES

PREPARATION: 20 MINUTES
EACH

*Mix up a batch of marinade and you're already partly done with dinner. Chicken can be prepared the night before, while beef can be marinated just a few hours before you pop the pan in the oven.*

*Simply pour the marinade over the meat, cover, and refrigerate, turning at least once so the liquid can soak through. For a super simple meal, just cook some baking potatoes with your meat and fix a salad.*

**GINGERY BARBECUE.** Fresh ginger really makes a difference!

½ **cup tamari soy sauce**
½ **cup oil**
**2 cloves garlic, minced**
¼ **cup honey**
**3 tablespoons freshly grated ginger**
**3 stalks chopped green onions**
**2 tablespoons sesame seeds**

**KOREAN MARINADE.** Heat mixture until boiling.

¼ **cup tamari soy sauce**
¼ **cup beef broth or water**
¼ **cup cider vinegar**
**Dash of honey, ginger, parsley**

# NACHOS WITH A FLOURISH

PREPARATION: 5 MINUTES
BAKING: 15 MINUTES
YIELD: 4–6 SERVINGS

**1 or 2 bags corn tortilla chips**
**1 small can refried beans**
   **(look for the vegetarian type without lard)**

2 cups grated cheddar cheese
1 small can sliced black olives (optional)
1 or 2 cups natural salsa
sour cream
avocado

Preheat the oven to 350°. Layer some of the chips in the bottom of a large pan and spoon on half the beans. Sprinkle on cheese and olives, then repeat the layers. End with chips and cheese. Bake for about 15 minutes or until the cheese bubbles. Top with salsa and sour cream, avocado, or whatever else sounds good. We often make two pans of nachos for dinner—one for the kids, with beans, chips, cheese, and a dribble of salsa, and another for the adults with chopped onion and jalapeño peppers.

# Nutty Buttermilk Chicken or Fish

PREPARATION: 25 MINUTES
BAKING: 1½ HOURS
YIELD: 1–4 SERVINGS

*More elaborate than ordinary oven-frying, but worth it!*

½ cup butter
1 cup buttermilk
1 egg, beaten
1 cup whole wheat flour
1 cup ground pecans or walnuts
⅓ cup sesame seeds
1 tablespoon paprika
1 3-pound chicken, cut up, or white fish pieces
⅔ cup pecan or walnut halves

Preheat the oven to 350°. Melt the butter in a large roasting pan in the oven and set aside. Combine the buttermilk and egg. In another bowl, mix the flour, ground nuts, seeds, and paprika. Coat the chicken in the buttermilk and then roll it in the flour mixture until it's covered. Put in pan, turning to cover all sides in butter. Sprinkle on the nut halves and bake for 1½ hours.

# Oven-Fried Chicken

PREPARATION: 10 MINUTES
BAKING: 45 MINUTES
YIELD: 4–6 SERVINGS

*Try to buy fresh, range-fed chicken.*

1 frying chicken, cut up
1 cup wheat germ
¼ teaspoon salt

¼ teaspoon basil
1 egg, beaten
⅓ cup milk

Preheat the oven to 325°. Mix the wheat germ, salt, and basil and put in a pie tin. Mix the egg and milk in a small soup bowl. Dip each chicken piece in the milk, then in the wheat germ, and place in a greased baking pan. Bake for 45 minutes or until pink juice doesn't run out of the chicken when it's poked. Serves four to six.

# Pumpkin Pot Stew

PREPARATION: 20 MINUTES
BAKING: 2 HOURS AND 20
MINUTES
YIELD: 4 OR MORE
SERVINGS

*After you've cut the top off a pumpkin and marveled at all the seeds, scrape out the pulp and you have a pumpkin pot.*

1 pumpkin, about 7 pounds
1 pound ground meat or cooked beans
2 cups chopped onion
3 tablespoons cooking oil
3 apples, cored and cut in large chunks
1 cup water or broth
½ cup raisins
Pinch of dried thyme

Preheat the oven to 350°. After removing the seeds and stringy pulp, place the pumpkin cut side down in a 13-inch by 9-inch by 2-inch deep baking dish. Pour ½ inch of water in the dish and bake for about 2 hours or until tender. Meanwhile, sauté the meat, onion, and apple until tender. Add the remaining ingredients and bring to a boil. Simmer until the pumpkin is done. Remove the pumpkin from the oven, drain water, and place it cut side up in the baking dish. Fill it with the meat or bean mixture and cover the top of the pumpkin with foil. Return it to the oven and bake it for 20 minutes or until hot. What a dramatic dinner—as you scoop out the filling, be sure to get some of the fragrant pumpkin flesh.

# Scalloped Potatoes With A Plus

PREPARATION: 20 MINUTES
BAKING: 1 HOUR
YIELD: 4 SERVINGS

½ pound ground turkey or beef
1 medium onion, chopped
2 tablespoons oil
4 potatoes, washed and dried

3 tablespoons whole wheat flour
3 cups milk
1 cup grated cheese

Preheat the oven to 350°. Cook the meat and onion in the oil until the meat is browned. Slice the potatoes very thin and layer them with the meat, cheese, and onions in a greased 2-quart casserole dish, sprinkling each layer with flour and ending with the potatoes. Heat the milk in the same pan you used to brown the meat. Pour it over the potatoes and bake for one hour.

# Slow-Cooker Beans

PREPARATION: 5 MINUTES
COOKING: 6–8 HOURS
YIELD: APPROXIMATELY 8 CUPS BEANS

*A convenient, nutritious way to use more beans in dishes.*

4 cups dried beans, such as pinto or kidney
6 cups hot water
Optional: ½ cup sliced onions
3 tablespoons catsup or molasses
1 tablespoon chili powder

Put all the ingredients in a slow-cooker and cook on high for six hours or on low for eight hours. Add more water if necessary. Cooked beans freeze well, so plan ahead for your next chili or taco feed!

# Tangy Lemon Fish

PREPARATION: 10 MINUTES
BAKING: 20 MINUTES
YIELD: 4 SERVINGS

1 pound white fish filets, such as halibut
1 tablespoon cooking oil
⅓ cup lemon juice
Pinch of parsley and grated onion

Preheat the oven to 325°. Separate the fish pieces and lay them in a single layer on an ungreased baking pan. Mix the remaining ingredients and pour them over the fish. Bake for 20 minutes or until the fish flakes easily with a fork. Toddlers love the delicate taste of fish, but be sure it's boned.

# Tofu Burgers or Cottage Cheese Burgers

PREPARATION: 10 MINUTES
BAKING: 1 HOUR
YIELD: 4 SERVINGS

6 eggs, beaten
1 cup chopped sunflower seeds or nuts
2 cups firm tofu, crumbled, or cottage cheese
1 cup dry whole wheat bread crumbs
¼ cup chopped onion
2 tablespoons butter for frying

Knead all the ingredients together and form into patties, or press into greased loaf pan for a meatloaf. Brown the patties in butter, or bake the meatloaf in a 350° oven for one hour.

# TUNA PATTIES

PREPARATION: 10 MINUTES
COOKING: 3–5 MINUTES
YIELD: 4 SERVINGS

*The flour coating makes a crunchy skin.*

**1 egg, beaten**
**1 cup cold mashed potatoes**
**1 small can tuna packed in water, drained well**
**¼ cup whole wheat flour**
**2 tablespoons butter or cooking oil**

Mix the egg, potatoes, and tuna, shape into patties and dust with flour. Melt the butter in a skillet and brown the patties, turning them just once. Serve plain, with tartar sauce (below), or as a sandwich filling.

**HOMEMADE TARTAR SAUCE:** Mix 1 tablespoon relish or chopped pickle, 1 cup mayonnaise, and 1 tablespoon vinegar. Chill.

# TWICE-BAKED POTATOES

PREPARATION: 20 MINUTES
BAKING: 1 HOUR PLUS 15 MINUTES
YIELD: 4 SERVINGS

*A "company" dinner item that kids love to have a hand in . . .*

**4 baking potatoes, scrubbed, then pricked with a fork**
**1 cup milk or less**
**1 onion or 4 green onions, chopped, sauteed or raw**
**Add-ins: grated cheese, chili, cooked pinto beans, leftover**
**    vegetables, or meat.**

Bake potatoes at 350° for one hour, or until they're soft when tested with a fork. Remove them from the oven and slice in half lengthwise. Scoop the soft potato insides into a bowl. Mash the potatoes, adding small amounts of milk, until creamy. Add cheese or other add-ins and refill the potato halves. Place them in a baking dish and reheat, or wrap them in foil for freezing and re-baking.

# WHOLE WHEAT PIZZA

PREPARATION: 20 MINUTES
BAKING: 15 MINUTES
YIELD: 4 OR MORE
SERVINGS

1 tablespoon yeast
1 cup warm water
1 teaspoon honey
1 tablespoon oil
4 cups whole wheat flour
2 cups natural spaghetti sauce
2 cups grated mozzarella or jack cheese
Optional toppings: sliced mushrooms, onions, green peppers,
    sausage, etc.

Preheat the oven to 400°. Dissolve the yeast in warm water for about five minutes. Add the honey and oil, then stir in the flour one cup at a time. Knead for about 10 minutes, adding more flour or water until the dough isn't sticky. Oil a pizza pan and roll or pat the dough to fit (save extra dough for pie crusts). Bake plain, without sauce or cheese, for 10 minutes. Then lower the heat to 350° and spread on the sauce and all the toppings but the cheese. Bake for five minutes and shut off the oven. Sprinkle on the cheese and melt it in the oven.

QUICK PIZZA FOR LUNCH. Spread sauce and cheese on a toasted English muffin and broil until bubbly.

# 12 BREADS

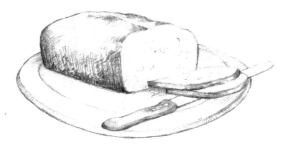

# CORN BREAD

*Kernels are the seeds of the corn plant.*

1 cup yellow cornmeal, whole grain
1 cup whole wheat flour
2 teaspoons baking powder
3 tablespoons oil
2 eggs, beaten
1 cup milk
Optional: ¼ cup raisins, grated cheese, nuts, chopped onions,
    sesame seeds

Preheat the oven to 350°. In a large bowl, mix the cornmeal, flour, and baking powder and set aside. In a small bowl, combine the oil, eggs, and milk. Add any optional ingredients and pour into dry mixture. Stir just until blended and pour batter into a greased 8-inch square pan. Bake for 30 minutes, or until the top springs back when you poke it.

# ELVES' BREAD

*Why does hot bread steam when we slice it? The water or milk in the batter changes to steam from being heated.*

1 cup whole wheat flour
½ teaspoon baking powder or soda
1 egg, beaten
½ cup yogurt, sour cream, or sour milk
¼ cup raisins
Optional: sprinkle of sesame or sunflower seeds on top

Preheat the oven to 375°. Stir together the flour and baking powder. Beat the egg and yogurt together in a separate bowl, then slowly stir into the dry mixture along with the raisins. Knead for about five minutes, then form the dough into a round, flat loaf. Place it on a greased baking sheet and slash the top about ½ inch deep. (Kids love to draw their initials or a swirly design on their loaf.) Bake for twenty minutes or until golden and crusty.

# SLOW-COOKER LOAF

PREPARATION: 15 MINUTES
COOKING: 3 HOURS
YIELD: 1 LOAF

*Yeast is a magic little plant. Once it's combined with warm liquid and a bit of sweetener, it breathes gas bubbles that make our bread taller and lighter. We knead our dough to spread those bubbles throughout the bread. What else do we use in cooking to make bubbles?*

1 tablespoon yeast
¼ cup warm water
1¼ cups warm milk
½ cup rolled oats
   or whole grain cornmeal
2 tablespoons oil or mellted butter
2 tablespoons molasses
1 egg, beaten

¼ cup wheat bran
   or wheat germ
3 to 4 cups whole
   wheat flour
½ cup sesame seeds

Optional: ½ teaspoon dill
   weed or chopped parsley

Preheat the cooker to high. Grease a one-pound metal coffee can or other bowl that will fit inside. Stir the yeast into the warm water and let it stand for five minutes. Add the milk, oats, oil, molasses, egg, and bran. Stir well, then add most of the flour (and the dill or parsley, if you want to) and knead with your hands (butter them first) until the dough is smooth and elastic. Add more water if the dough is too dry, or add water if it gets sticky. Put the dough in the can, sprinkle seeds on top, and cover it loosely with foil. Put crumpled aluminum foil or a trivet on the bottom of the cooker and pour in ¾ cup of water. Then place the can of bread on the trivet, cover the cooker, and bake for three hours. Turn out and slice. Since this loaf steams rather than oven-bakes, it won't brown. Delicious!

# Raisin Bran Muffins

*This is a great-tasting, high-fiber breakfast treat that kids love.*

2½ cups whole grain raisin bran cereal, unsweetened
2½ cups whole wheat flour
4 teaspoons baking powder
4 eggs, beaten
½ cup cooking oil, preferably cold-pressed
1 cup molasses (or ½ cup honey and ½ cup molasses)
**Optional: we like to add ½ cup extra raisins**

Preheat the oven to 350°. Combine the cereal, flour, and baking powder in a large bowl and set it aside. In a separate bowl, blend the eggs, oil, and molasses. Mix all the ingredients together, stirring just until the batter is thoroughly moist. Fill greased muffin cups ⅔ full and bake for 25 to 30 minutes.

# 13 BEVERAGES

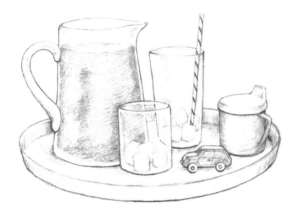

# BLENDER FRUIT PUNCH

PREPARATION: 5 MINUTES
YIELD: 2 SERVINGS

*Where are the seeds in a strawberry? An orange? Pineapple? Banana?*

**1 cup thawed unsweetened pineapple juice concentrate**
**3 oranges, peeled, seeded, cut in pieces**
**2 cups chopped strawberries, unsweetened**
**1 cup or more club soda or mineral water**

Puree all the fruit and the pineapple juice in a blender. When you're ready to serve it, pour the drink over ice in a punch bowl and add bubbly soda or mineral water at the last minute.

# CRANBERRY APPLE GROG

PREPARATION: 5 MINUTES
YIELD: 10 SERVINGS

*This is best when made the day before.*

**1 bottle of unsweetened apple juice: 44 oz.**
**1 bottle of unsweetened cranberry juice: 44 oz.**
**2 cups raisins**
**2 oranges, sliced and studded with whole cloves**
**3 cinnamon sticks**

Combine all the ingredients and let stand. The next day, bring to a boil and simmer for 1 hour or keep warm in a slow-cooker. Serve hot.

# HOT CAROB DRINK

PREPARATION: 10 MINUTES
YIELD: 4 SERVINGS

**4 tablespoons sifted carob powder**
**3 tablespoons honey or light molasses**
**5 cups whole milk**
**2 teaspoons pure vanilla extract**
**Optional: whipped cream**

Mix the carob powder, honey, and one cup of the milk in a small saucepan over medium heat, stirring constantly. When all the ingredients are liquid and hot, stir in the remaining milk and heat through. Just before serving, add the vanilla and ladle the hot drink into mugs. Top with whipped cream if desired.

# ICED HERBAL SUN TEA

*A cool refresher without caffeine*

**1 herbal tea bag per serving**
**1 cup water per serving**
**Sun!**

Put the tea bags and water in a large glass jar and set it outside or in a window that gets lots of sunshine. Check the tea often—the darker the tea, the stronger its taste. When it's well-steeped, chill and serve over ice cubes.

# Kids' FAVORITE DRINKS

YIELD: 2 SERVINGS

To ½ cup sparkling mineral water, add ¼ cup lemon juice and ¼ cup unsweetened apple or grape juice.

YIELD: 4 SERVINGS

For imitation ice smoothies, blend 1 small can frozen unsweetened grape juice concentrate with ½ cup water; then add 8 ice cubes and whirl in a blender. Serve in paper cups.

# Lemonade

PREPARATION: 10 MINUTES
YIELD: 2 SERVINGS

*Why do we love citrus fruits, like lemons, oranges, and grapefruit? Maybe because they are loaded with vitamin C. Without it, we'd get scurvy, a disease that was once common on ships and in prisons where people didn't have fresh fruit and vegetables.*

**2 cups water**
**1 or 2 lemons, depending on your taste**
**1 or 2 teaspoons honey**

Put the water in a pan and heat it to boiling. Turn off the heat. Cut the lemon in half and pinch out any seeds. Squeeze the lemon juice into the hot water and drop the lemon rind in, too. Stir in the honey until it dissolves and pour the liquid into a pitcher. Chill and remove lemon rinds before serving in glasses with ice.

# Smells-So-Good Cider

PREPARATION: 5 MINUTES
COOKING: 2 HOURS OR 20
    MINUTES
YIELD: 6 SERVINGS

**2 quarts apple juice, unsweetened and preferably unfiltered**
**1 whole orange, studded with cloves**
**3 sticks cinnamon**
**Pinch of allspice, ginger**

**SLOW-COOKER METHOD:** Pour the juice into the cooker, then add the orange and spice. Cook on low for 2 hours and serve warm.

**STOVE-TOP METHOD:** Mix all the ingredients in a large pan and bring to a boil over medium heat. Cover, reduce heat, and simmer for 20 minutes. Serve it now, or let the flavors blend overnight: cool and strain, then refrigerate. Reheat before serving.

# Wallace's Breakfast Drink

PREPARATION: 5 MINUTES
YIELD: 2 LARGE SERVINGS

*The nutrients in this fast, easy drink are in their natural state and easily absorbed.*

**12 ounces juice (unfiltered apple is good)**
**2 whole bananas, peeled**
**1 tablespoon brewer's yeast**
**1 tablespoon flaked spirulina**
**1 tablespoon soy protein powder**
**Optional: 1 tablespoon natural peanut butter**
    **Peaches, pineapple, berries, or other favorite fruits**
    **Calcium, magnesium powder**

Put all the ingredients in a blender and whirl until smooth. Add the liquid vitamins for a highly nutritious drink.

# 14 SWEET STUFF AND TREATS

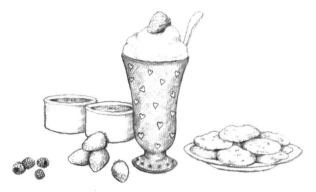

# 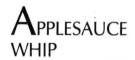PPLESAUCE WHIP

PREPARATION: 10 MINUTES
YIELD: 4 SERVINGS

*An easy, firm dessert.*

**2 teaspoons gelatin**　　　　　　**1 cup unsweetened applesauce**
**1 cup unsweetened apple juice**

Dissolve the gelatin in the juice and add the applesauce. Chill until the mixture is runny, then whip it until it's fluffy and about double in size. Chill again before serving.

**FOR OLDER TASTES:** top with yogurt or unsweetened whipped cream.


# CAROB-COATED APPLES

PREPARATION: 30 MINUTES
YIELD: 8 PIECES

*Since melted carob hardens so quickly, you have to have everything set up beforehand. Have a clean plate and waxed paper near the stove for the cooling apples.*

**8 medium-size apples**
**8 wooden popsicle sticks**
**1 pound carob, in chips or cut into small pieces**
**Optional: 1 cup roasted peanuts, chopped**
**　　　　　 1 cup toasted coconut, shredded**

Put the sticks into the stem end of the apples and place everything within easy reach of the stove. Then melt the carob over simmering water in a double boiler, stirring occasionally. As soon as the carob is completely melted, roll an apple in it until it is covered and then hold it over the pan for a few seconds so any extra can drip back. If you like, hold the apple over the plate and sprinkle the nuts or coconut over it. Let cool on the waxed paper, stick up, while you quickly dip the remaining apples. Children love to help make this recipe, and often prefer to use a spoon to sprinkle nuts over the carob-coated apple.

# CAROB MOUSSE

*Use a double boiler whenever you melt carob.*

**1 pound carob chips, unsweetened or mint flavored**
**6 eggs, separated**

Melt the carob in a double boiler; remove it from the heat but leave it over the hot water. Beat the egg yolks and stir them into the carob; then remove the carob from over the water. Beat the egg whites until they're stiff. Carefully fold in the egg whites. Chill at least three hours.

# CHARNA'S CREAMY CAROB CANDY

**½ cup honey**
**½ cup light molasses**
**1 cup natural peanut butter**
**1 cup sifted carob powder**
**2 teaspoons vanilla**
**8 ounces cream cheese**
**Optional: ½ cup chopped nuts**

Cook the honey, molasses, and peanut butter in a small pan until they melt together. Stir this mixture often to make sure it doesn't burn. Then remove it from the heat and add the other ingredients. Mix well and spread into a greased 8-inch square pan. Chill for at least one hour before you cut it into bite-size pieces. Enjoy! Any leftovers must be refrigerated because of the cream cheese.

# Drugstore Egg Custard

PREPARATION: 10 MINUTES
BAKING: 30 MINUTES
YIELD: 6 SERVINGS

*A handy protein food.*

7 eggs, beaten
⅔ cup light honey
2 teaspoons pure vanilla
1½ quarts hot milk
Topping: ½ cup bran flakes or coconut
    dash of cinnamon or nutmeg

Preheat the oven to 325°. Mix the egg, honey, and vanilla until they're smooth. Beat in the hot milk. Pour this liquid into a 9-inch by 13-inch pan and bake over hot water for 30 minutes or until firm. Sprinkle on the topping before or after baking.

# Flaky Almond Balls

PREPARATION: 15 MINUTES
CHILL: 1 HOUR
BAKING: 10 MINUTES
YIELD: 48 COOKIES

*Split an almond in half and look at the tiny start of a new almond plant.*

2 cups oil
6 tablespoons light honey
4 cups whole wheat pastry flour
2 cups almonds, ground or finely chopped
2 teaspoons almond extract

Preheat the oven to 400°. Beat the oil and honey together in a large bowl. Add the remaining ingredients and stir until the batter is well blended. Put the bowl in your refrigerator and chill for at least one hour or until the batter has slightly stiffened. Now grease your hands and shape the dough into walnut-size balls. Place these on a lightly greased cookie sheet and bake for about 10 minutes.

# FRUIT JUICE FINGER FOOD

PREPARATION: 10 MINUTES
CHILL: 1 HOUR

*Gelatin is a powdery protein that soaks up liquid and makes mixtures harden. We can buy it in ready-to-use granules, or make it from bones boiled a long time.*

½ **tablespoon gelatin**
⅛ **cup cold water**
⅓ **cup boiling water**
½ **cup unsweetened juice, such as peach or apple**

Soak the gelatin in the cold water, then dissolve it in the boiling water. Add the juice and pour this mixture into an ice cube tray or small mold. Chill until set.

**FOR OLDER TASTES:** Add diced fruit, such as apples, melon, raisins, grapes, and so forth.


# FUDGEY SICKLES

PREPARATION: 15 MINUTES
YIELD: 6 SERVINGS

**1 cup thawed juice concentrate (apple or pear-grape is good)**
**2 teaspoons butter**
**6 tablespoons carob powder**
**3 cups whole milk**

In a medium saucepan, boil the juice concentrate and butter, then stir in the carob powder and let cool. Beat in the milk and then pour the hot liquid into freezer cups with sticks as handles. Our kids love to use an ice cube tray with toothpicks.

# 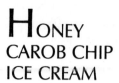ONEY CAROB CHIP ICE CREAM

PREPARATION: 15 MINUTES
CHILL: 7 HOURS
YIELD: 1 QUART

*Too rich for a daily food, but nice on a hot summer day.*

**3 eggs, beaten**
**½ cup honey**
**2 cups cream (or milk)**
**2 cups milk**
**2 teaspoons pure vanilla extract**
**⅔ cup unsweetened carob chips (try mint flavored)**

Beat the eggs and milk together in a large saucepan. Add the honey and cook over low heat, stirring constantly until thickened. The mixture should smoothly coat your spoon. Cool, then add the cream and vanilla. Refrigerate overnight. Next, follow the directions for your electric ice cream maker, and add the carob chips halfway through the freezing process.

# 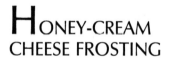ONEY-CREAM CHEESE FROSTING

PREPARATION: 5 MINUTES
YIELD: ENOUGH FOR ONE
8-INCH SQUARE CAKE
OR 12 CUPCAKES

**8 ounces cream cheese, softened**
**3 or more tablespoons light honey**

With an electric mixer (or many hand strokes), beat the cream cheese and honey together until all the lumps are gone and the frosting is spreadable. You may need to add more honey if you like a thinner frosting. Refrigerate or use immediately on cooled cake.

# 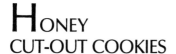Honey CUT-OUT COOKIES

PREPARATION: 20 MINUTES
BAKING: 10 MINUTES
YIELD: ABOUT 24 COOKIES

*Why do some honeys taste different? The flavor depends on which flowers the bees choose for lunch.*

**¼ cup light honey**
**¼ cup light molasses**
**½ cup melted butter**
**2 cups whole wheat flour**
**1 teaspoon baking soda**
**1 teaspoon cinnamon**
**¼ teaspoon allspice**

Preheat the oven to 350°. Cream the honey, molasses, the butter. Sift the remaining ingredients and blend them with the honey mixture. Chill the dough overnight, then divide it into thirds for easy rolling. Roll out onto a lightly floured or greased surface. (Our children prefer to butter their hands and pat the dough until it's thin and flat.) Use your favorite cookie cutters or form letters, numbers, and other designs. Place these on a lightly buttered cookie sheet and bake for about 10 minutes. Remove the cookies from the sheet quickly and let them cool before you decorate them.

TO DECORATE: Use cream cheese frosting, raisins, nuts, and so on. You can also put a single piece of macaroni in the top of each cookie before baking. After it cools, a string or ribbon may be drawn through the macaroni so that the cookie can be a necklace, tree ornament, or window hanger.

# Honey Granola Cookies

PREPARATION: 15 MINUTES
BAKING: 10 MINUTES
YIELD: 24 COOKIES

**1 cup butter**
**½ cup honey**
**1 teaspoon vanilla**
**1 cup whole wheat pastry flour**
**1 egg**
**½ cup each shredded coconut and chopped nuts**
**3 cups rolled oats**
**1 cup raisins**

Preheat the oven to 350°. Melt the butter and stir in the honey until they're smooth. Add the other ingredients and mix well. Drop the batter a teaspoonful at a time onto a greased baking sheet and bake for 10 minutes.

# Instant Sherbet

PREPARATION: 5 MINUTES

**1 cup frozen fruit (berries, peaches, bananas)**
**¼ cup apple juice concentrate, thawed**

Splash some juice concentrate onto the fruit and swirl it in a blender until smooth, adding more liquid if necessary. If your fruit is too bitter, add a spoonful of honey. Serve immediately as a slushy treat, or pour into little cups and freeze for later.

# IRISH GINGERBREAD

PREPARATION: 15 MINUTES
BAKING: 45 MINUTES
YIELD: 8 SERVINGS

2 cups whole wheat flour, sifted
2 teaspoons baking soda
1½ teaspoons cinnamon
1 teaspoon ginger
½ cup butter, softened
⅓ cup honey

2 eggs, beaten
1 cup molasses
½ cup old-fashioned oats,
   softened in water
   and drained
1 cup hot water

Preheat the oven to 350°. Mix the flour, baking soda, cinnamon, and ginger in a large bowl and set aside. Cream the butter with the honey and eggs, beating well. Add the molasses and then the dry ingredients, stirring until fully blended. Mix in the oatmeal and then the hot water until the batter is smooth. Pour into a greased 8-inch square baking pan and bake for 45 minutes.


# MAIREAD'S FROZEN TREATS

PREPARATION: 10 MINUTES
CHILL: 2 HOURS

1 cup seedless melon (such as cantaloupe, honeydew, or
   watermelon), chopped
1 cup unsweetened juice or fruit punch
½ cup water

Put all the ingredients into a blender and whirl until smooth. Pour into an ice cube tray and place in a freezer. After about an hour, check to see if the liquid is firm enough to stand a toothpick in the center of each cube. Continue freezing for another hour or until the cubes are hard enough to remove and enjoy!

# MAKE YOUR OWN SHAKE

PREPARATION: 10 MINUTES
YIELD: 1 SHAKE

*What is powdered milk? It's milk particles that have been air-dried to take out most of the moisture. Instant milk powder is yellow and grainy, and non-instant looks like fine white face powder.*

**Chopped ice (give each child two ice cubes in a plastic sandwich bag and let him flail with a hammer. FUN!)**
**Small unbreakable jar or container with snug lid**
**6 tablespoons instant powdered milk**
**8 tablespoons of your favorite fruit juice**

Put ½ cup chopped ice into the jar or container. Add the milk powder and fruit juice. Screw on the top and shake until the powdered milk dissolves. If you have a really tight lid, let your child sit on the floor and roll the jar around with her feet!

# MAPLE SNOW (OR ICE CUBE) PUDDING

PREPARATION: 5 MINUTES
YIELD: 2–3 SERVINGS

**2 cups of clean, new snow (or 2 trays of ice cubes)**
**1 cup pure maple syrup, heated**

If you're using ice cubes, wrap them in a towel and smash them with a hammer. (Kids love to do this!) Put the "snow" in cups and cover it with warm maple syrup.

# PEACH COBBLER

*Also delicious with mixed peaches and blueberries.*

3 tablespoons cornstarch or arrowroot powder
1 can unsweetened apple juice concentrate, thawed: 12 ounces
¼ teaspoon pure almond extract
4 cups sliced peaches, unsweetened
1½ cups whole wheat flour
2¼ teaspoons baking powder
4 tablespoons melted butter
2 tablespoons chopped almonds

Preheat the oven to 400°. In a medium saucepan, mix the cornstarch with 1 cup of the juice concentrate and the almond extract. Heat, stirring often, for about five minutes until the mixture thickens. Add the peaches, coat them with the glaze, and spoon them into an 8-inch square pan. In a small bowl, mix the flour and baking powder. Add the butter and the remaining ½ cup of apple juice concentrate. Stir in the nuts and spoon the batter over the fruit. Bake for 30 minutes.


# PEACHY-KEEN SUNDAE

Frozen raspberries, unsweetened
Honey vanilla ice cream
Fresh or canned peach halves, unsweetened
Sliced almonds or other favorite nuts

Mash the raspberries or whirl them in a blender until they're smooth. Put one scoop of ice cream into a dish, top it with a peach, and smother the whole thing in raspberry sauce. Top with nuts and enjoy!

# PEANUT BUTTER COOKIES FOR A CROWD

PREPARATION: 20 MINUTES
BAKING: 10 MINUTES PER
  BATCH
YIELD: 5 DOZEN COOKIES

1 cup butter or ½ cup butter and ½ cup oil
1 cup peanut butter or other nut butter
1 cup honey or ½ cup honey and ½ cup molasses
2 eggs, beaten
1 teaspoon pure vanilla extract
2 cups whole wheat flour
2 teaspoons baking soda
½ cup non-instant dry milk powder
  or ¾ cup instant dry milk powder
Options: ½ cup carob chips, sunflower or sesame seeds,
  wheat germ, rolled oats, nuts, dried fruit

Preheat the oven to 350°. Cream the butter, peanut butter, and honey. Add the egg and vanilla, beating well. Stir in the remaining ingredients and drop a teaspoonful at a time onto a lightly greased cookie sheet. Flatten with a fork dipped into water. Bake for 10 minutes or until golden.


# QUICK FRUIT ICE CREAM

PREPARATION: 5 MINUTES
YIELD: 1 HEFTY SERVING

*Teething toddlers especially love this icy treat.*

**Frozen, peeled fruit (2 bananas, 2 peaches, 6 apricots, or your favorites)**

Whirl the fruit in a blender or food processor until smooth. Also wonderful with a dash of vanilla or orange peel.

# Tropical Carob Bites

PREPARATION: 20 MINUTES
YIELD: 8 SMALL HELPINGS

**1 pound carob chips**
**2 cups unsweetened coconut, shredded and toasted**

Melt the carob over simmering water in a double boiler. Stir in the coconut and mix well. Drop a tablespoonful at a time onto waxed paper and let cool. These are great lunchbox treats if you pack them with something cold so the carob doesn't melt.

# Whole Wheat Carob Chip Cookies

PREPARATION: 15 MINUTES
BAKING: 10 MINUTES
YIELD: 24 COOKIES

*Carob is dark brown like chocolate, but doesn't contain sugar, caffeine, or fat.*

**¾ cup honey**
**¾ cup molasses**
**1 cup butter**
**1 teaspoon vanilla**
**2 eggs, beaten**
**2½ cups whole wheat pastry flour**
**1½ teaspoons baking soda**
**12 ounces unsweetened carob chips**
    **(or try mint-flavored or date sugar chips)**
**Optional: 1 cup chopped walnuts**

Preheat the oven to 375°. Cream the honey, molasses, and butter. Add the vanilla and eggs. Mix well. In a separate bowl, stir together the flour and baking soda, then add them to the honey mixture. Add the carob chips (and optional walnuts) and blend well. Drop a tablespoonful at a time onto a lightly greased cookie sheet. Bake for about 10 minutes.

# YOUR OWN PEANUT BUTTER CUPS

PREPARATION: 25 MINUTES
YIELD: 8 SERVINGS

*A look-alike candy.*

**1 cup natural peanut butter, creamy**
**3 tablespoons honey**
**1 pound carob, melted**

Mix the peanut butter with the honey. On waxed paper, drop teaspoons of carob to make 2-inch circles. Spoon a bit of peanut butter in the center of each circle and spread more carob over the entire piece. Cool. Our three children would gladly eat all of these as soon as they cooled. For guests, count on this recipe serving eight.

# 15 ALPHABET RECIPES

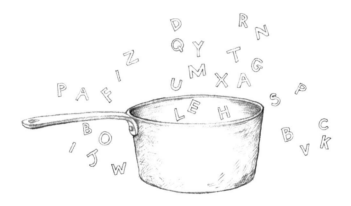

**C**OOKING CAN be a great learning tool that's both friendly and sharing. As helpers, children develop motor skills, explore social interactions, and even learn academic basics such as math (measuring) and phonics (recipe reading).

Younger chefs are especially thrilled to see letters they know in whatever they're doing. Here are some super simple ideas for quick cooking (even with a crowd) that also use the alphabet. To really jazz up the session, try drawing out the recipe on large cards and underlining the fun major letter.

**A**pplesauce from a Blender. Wash five large apples. Quarter, core, and peel them, then pop a few at a time into the blender along with a cup of water. Add one teaspoon cinnamon and whirl until mushy. Serve in a cup. YUM!

**B**utter from Muscle Power. Put some cream (without preservatives) into a baby food jar or any other see-through container with a tight lid. Add a dash of salt, cap tightly, and shake. (Friends can really help here.) When you see yellow chunks of butter, pour off the buttermilk and spread.

**C**razy Carrot Cars. Wash a carrot and a stalk of celery. Cut the celery into 2-inch sticks and the carrot into round "wheels." Stick a wheel onto each end of two toothpicks and lay a celery car on top. You can fill your car with peanut butter, cream cheese, or raisins.

**D**iggety-Dog Dip. Boil five no-nitrate hot dogs in water until they're cooked. Slice them into small pieces and put the pieces in a blender along with ½ cup mayonnaise, one tablespoon mustard, and ½ cup chopped pickles or relish. Whirl until smooth and serve with whole grain crackers. A fun way to eat protein!

**E**gg in a Nest. Put a slice of whole wheat bread on a flat surface and use a small glass to cut out a circle in the center. Melt two tablespoons of butter in a skillet and fry both pieces of bread, turning them over to brown both sides. Break an egg into the hole and cook gently until it's done. You can fit the cutout circle atop the egg as a hat.

**F**ruit Leather. *Cooking method:* Choose any fruit (or fruit combination such as peaches, apricots, or pears) and cut off any bruises before putting it in a large pot. Cook gently, stirring occasionally, and add honey if desired. When the fruit looks like a thick puree, spread it evenly on cookie sheets lined with waxed paper. Dry in a slow oven for about an hour, or sun-dry, covering the pan with cheese-cloth if necessary to keep away insects. When the sheets are dry, cut them into strips, roll them up, and store in an air-tight jar. So much better than the corn-syrupy artificially colored supermarket stuff!! *No-cook method:* Take two cups dried fruit and run twice through the fine blade of fruit grinder. Put some of the ground fruit between two sheets of waxed paper and flatten with a rolling pin until the fruit layer is very thin. Peel the fruit leather from the paper, or you can roll it up to eat later. A great lunchbox addition.

**G**ranola. In a large bowl, mix three cups rolled oats with one cup each of wheat germ and sesame seeds. Put ½ cup oil, ½ cup honey, and two teaspoons vanilla in a large baking pan and heat in a 275° oven until liquid. Add the oat mixture and stir to coat evenly. Bake for an hour, stirring every 15 minutes. When it's dry to your liking, break up any large lumps and add nuts, raisins, dates, or coconut. Store in an air-tight container. Great for camping and snacking.

**H**ard-(or Soft-) Boiled Eggs. Put eggs in a pan and fill with cold water. Turn the heat to high and cook until the water boils. Turn down the heat and cook fifteen minutes for hard-boiled eggs and three minutes for soft. Drain the eggs and put them under cold running water to keep the shells from sticking when you peel them. Kids really love hard-boiled eggs if they can use a fancy slicer to cut the eggs with straight or scalloped edges.

**I**nstant Clay. DON'T EAT! Mix four cups of flour with one cup salt in a bowl. Add one tablespoon oil and 1½ cups water, using your hands to get it good and gooey. Mix for about five minutes and use within the next few hours before it hardens. You can use a rolling pin and cookie cutters for nice designs. Bake at 350° for an hour, and paint for decorations. This clay makes sturdy Christmas tree ornaments, paperweights, and dinosaurs!

**J**elly Fingers. A healthy finger food that won't melt. Put one cup water in a pan and sprinkle three tablespoons of unflavored gelatin on top. When you see the gelatin soften, turn the heat on gently and stir until it dissolves. Add six ounces of a thawed juice concentrate, such as apple, grape, or orange, and pour into an 8-inch square pan. Chill to set and cut into fingers or other fun shapes.

**K**ugel. Cook ¼ pound whole wheat noodles until tender, then drain. Add two beaten eggs, one cup milk, ½ cup yogurt or sour cream, one cup raisins, one teaspoon vanilla, and a dash of cinnamon. Melt three tablespoons butter in a large baking pan and spread in the noodle mixture. Bake at 350° for about 45 minutes.

**L**etter Pretzels. Dissolve one tablespoon yeast in 1½ cups warm water. Add one tablespoon honey, one teaspoon salt, and two cups whole wheat flour. Beat until smooth, then slowly add two more cups of flour and knead. When the dough is firm and stretchy, put it back in the bowl, cover it with a towel, and let it rise for an hour, if desired. Then punch it down, divide it into pieces, and let everyone roll their own ropes and make letters. Put all finished pretzels on a greased baking sheet and let them rest for twenty minutes. Brush with beaten egg white and sprinkle with salt. Bake at 425° for fifteen minutes.

**M**elted Tuna and Cheese Sandwich. Mix a small can of tuna with three tablespoons mayonnaise. Add some chopped onion and relish, if you like. Put a scoop on top of the English muffin halves and top with a slice of cheese. Toast under broiler until the cheese melts, and garnish with tomato bits or sprouts. Serve hot.

**N**atural Food Colorings. Use these to paint toast, color eggs, tint bath water, and so on. For *army-green*, use red onion skins. For *brown*, use coffee. For *blue*, use blueberries. For *lavender*, use blackberries or violets. For *green*, use spinach or carrot tops. For *red*, use beets. For yellow, use *yellow* onion skins. Put whatever dyeing material you choose into a non-aluminum pot, cover with water, and boil until the color is dark. You can crush the materials for more intense color. Strain and use hot if you're dyeing eggs. Children who are allergic to artificial colorings can safely tint cupcake frostings and other goodies with these.

**O**nion Soup While You Sleep. Slice five large onions into rings. Put the rings in a slow cooker and cover them with about eight cups of chicken or beef broth. Cover and cook on low for twenty-four hours. Ladle the soup into oven-proof bowls and top with a thick slice of whole grain bread. Cover the bread with Swiss or Jack cheese and broil until the cheese melts.

**P**ow-Wow Beef Jerky. Trim any fat off two pounds of flank steak. Cut the steak in half, then cut against the grain into strips about five inches long and ¼ inch thick. Put the meat in a bowl and marinate for thirty minutes in ½ cup tamari soy sauce with two cloves minced garlic. Drain and arrange strips in a single layer in a drain rack set in a large baking pan. Bake at 150° overnight, or for twelve hours. When the meat has dried, drain it on paper towels and store in an airtight jar.

**Q**uick, No-Cook Peanut Butter Balls. Stir together ½ cup natural peanut butter and ½ cup honey. Then add one cup dry milk powder, preferably non-instant. Here's where the mucky fun begins: let everyone knead the mixture, adding more milk powder or honey if needed, until you can shape the dough into walnut-size balls. You can roll the balls in coconut or chopped nuts, or fashion them into little mice. Serve immediately or chill. A real favorite that's also a protein bonanza.

**R**aisins on a Log. Break off several celery stalks and wash them well. Pat them dry and spread peanut butter or cream cheese in the grooves. Don't eat yet! Now make your own designs with raisins, chopped nuts, or seeds on top of the peanut butter. You can even make it "snow" with coconut. This is good for a snack or a group activity. My daughter's Brownie troop goes bonkers decorating celery and crackers with a variety of good stuff.

**S**eeds From Scratch. Next time you carve out a pumpkin or cook a squash, save the seeds and try to guess how many there are. After you count them and see which guess was closest, mix the seeds in a bowl with three tablespoons water and four tablespoons tamari soy sauce. Oil a baking sheet and spread out the seeds. Bake at 350° for about ten to fifteen minutes, and nibble at will.

**T**omato Tidbits. Pick out large, firm cherry tomatoes and wash well. Carefully slice off the top (where the stem was) and scoop out the insides. You can save the pulp and seeds to combine with cottage cheese, then spoon back inside the tomato shells. Top with salt or sesame seeds and gobble up! You can spice them up with chopped onion, cheese, and other fillings.

**U**nbelievable Squash Muffins. To ⅔ cup cooked squash, add one cup milk, three tablespoons honey or molasses, and one beaten egg. In a separate bowl, sift together ⅔ cup whole wheat flour and three teaspoons baking powder. Add to the squash mixture along with one teaspoon melted butter. Spoon into greased muffin tins (each should be ⅔ full) and bake at 350° for twenty-five minutes.

**V**ery Veggie Soup. Wash your favorite vegetables, such as potatoes, carrots, mushrooms, and celery. Cut them into bite-size pieces and place them in a large pot along with eight cups of chicken stock or water. Bring to a boil and simmer for thirty mintues or longer, then add cooked chicken bits (optional) and cooked rice or noodles. Heat through and ladle into soup bowls.

**W**hole Wheat Tortillas (Chapatis). Mix together six cups whole wheat flour, 1½ teaspoons salt, and ½ teaspoon baking powder. Add ½ cup oil and about 1¼ cups warm water, kneading to make a soft dough that sticks together. Form about twenty balls and let them rest for about twenty minutes. You can then use a roller or your hands to pat the balls into thin circles, adding more flour if necessary. Cook on an ungreased skillet, flipping each tortilla until both sides are dotted with brown specks. Use for enchiladas, melt cheese in the middle for quesadillas, or cut into triangles and fry in oil for your own tortilla chips.

**X**-Tra Easy Party Punch. Pour equal amounts of unsweetened apple juice or cider and unsweetened cranberry juice in a large punch bowl. Pour in a can of thawed orange or apple juice concentrate. You can add some mineral water for fizzy bubbles.

**Y**ogurt Popsicles. Put into a blender two cups yogurt (plain if you're adding your own fruit), about six ounces thawed frozen juice concentrate (or 1½ cups unsweetened fruit juice), and a dash of vanilla. Throw in some fresh fruit like peaches or banana. Whirl everything until smooth, then pour into small paper cups and stick in the freezer. Eat as sundaes or put a plastic spoon in as a handle before the popsicle is completely frozen.

**Z**ucchini Cake. In a large bowl, mix one cup whole wheat flour, two teaspoons baking powder, and one teaspoon cinnamon. Stir in ⅓ cup oil, ⅓ cup honey, two beaten eggs, one cup grated zucchini, and ½ cup chopped nuts. You may also add up to ½ cup crushed, unsweetened pineapple. Pour the batter into a greased 8-inch square pan and bake at 350° for twenty to thirty minutes. This cake is moist as is, or frost it with a cream cheese and honey frosting.

# 16 PARTY IDEAS, MONTH BY MONTH

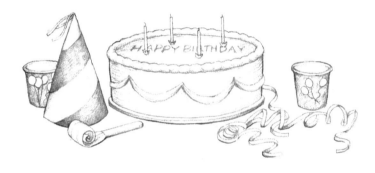

**W**HETHER YOU'RE cooking with one toddler or a whole class of kids, you'll find that everybody loves to prepare for a theme party. It's even more fun if everyone gets to help with the decorations and refreshments. This can play down the emphasis of party games and gifts.

Here are some ideas for get-togethers for children of all ages. Some of our most successful parties have been spur-of-the-moment, non-birthday celebrations. Just try to remember that kids are happiest with simple ideas, especially if they get to have a hand in the festivities. Check in the index for the page numbers of the recipes marked with an asterisk (*).

# September

**Autumn Party.** Decorate with a harvest theme—lots of golds and browns. Maybe have everybody bring some colored leaves and make nature collages. If you have a yard with trees, kids can rake leaves and jump in them. Talk about the harvests and prepare some apple treats, such as:

> **Surprise Apple Pancakes\*, topped with Applesauce from a Blender\***

**Back-to-School Computer Party.** Use high-tech decorations and computer-printed invitations. Beforehand, bake a double recipe of:
> **Zucchini Cake\* in a 9-inch by 13-inch pan**
> **Honey Cream Cheese Frosting\***

Decorate the cake to look like a computer-keyboard, using small alphabet letters cut from index cards to look like keys. If you have a computer, take turns playing games while others play "Pin the Letter on the Computer." Or they can play charades by making alphabet letters with their bodies.

# October

**Halloween Party.** Decorate with black and orange. Throw a costume party where everyone gets a prize and plays games like bob-for-apples. For dinner have something fun and easy like:
> **Bucket of Brains (spaghetti)**
> **Skeleton Bones (carrot sticks)**
> **Seeds from Scratch\***
> **Witches Brew (apple juice with a few pieces of dry ice tossed in for bubbles)**

# November 🎉

**Pioneer Party.** Celebrate with a mini-feast and talk about the Pilgrims and Indians. Your child may be surprised to learn what the first Thanksgiving foods really were! Make up your own rain dance and cut out Pilgrim hats or Indian feathers to wear. Make:

**Pow-Wow Beef Jerky***
**Corn Bread***, served with honey
**Butter from Muscle Power***
**Homemade Country Fries***
**Cranberry Sauce**
**Turkey slices (optional)**
**Cranberry juice, diluted with sparkling mineral water**

# December 🎉

**Holiday Cookie Swap.** This morning party is a yearly tradition for many of our friends. Host it as close to the holidays as possible so the treats will be fresh for gift-giving. First, figure out how many people want to swap cookies. Suppose six people are coming: they each should bring six dozen cookies (or more if lots of kids will sample). Each dozen should be wrapped individually with the cookie recipe attached. Once everybody arrives, each contributor gets a dozen of everybody else's cookies. The extra dozen from each person's own recipe is laid out (along with the other extras) for tasting. For a more meaningful holiday party, make it into a "can-share" with everybody contributing some canned food to a food basket for a local charity. We're never sure which is more fun, getting together for a holiday party, bringing home lots of delicious cookies, or the leisurely morning of sampling treats and sipping Smells-So-Good Cider*. Some parents may want to establish some guidelines first, so that everybody will bake reasonably healthy cookies. This party works well in a schoolroom setting, too. For larger groups, cut down the amount of cookies each person brings. You might have each student bring thirty bags of two cookies each, for example. This is a good way to amass cookies before a Christmas caroling party.

# January 🎉

**Winter Brunch.** Terrific just before an ice-skating party or a whale-watching group. Brunch is much more fun than the ho-hum lunch sandwich, and there are so many different items to try. If you're planning on pleasing a crowd, try giving each child something to contribute (even if it's being the Official Counter of Stirs) and make:

**Eggs, soft-boiled or scrambled**
**Almond Coffee Cake***
**Fresh orange or graperuit juice**
**Hot tea**
**Hot Carob Drink***

# February 🎉

**Valentine's Day Party.** Decorate with red and white. Make your own valentines with lace remnants or buttons on red construction paper, white paper doilies, and glitter. Serve cream of tomato soup during crafts. Everybody can run off steam during games. You can make:

**Honey Cut-Out Cookies***

before or after game time with heart-shaped cookie cutters.

# March 🎉

**Saint Patrick's Day Dinner.** Decorate with greens and shamrocks. Have everybody bring their favorite green vegetable to cut and put into boiling water for:

**Very Veggie Soup* (simmer during party games)**
**Slow Cooker Loaf* (with some green herbs)**
**Zucchini Cake***

Children love to play "Catch the Button" while waiting for the soup to finish cooking. Make paper cups or cones of green cardboard and decorate with shamrocks or pipe cleaners. Use large green buttons and pair off children so each has a partner. One child holds a cup while the other tosses buttons into the cup. Each child takes turns catching the buttons, and the one with the most catches is the winner. (Winners get to eat first!)

# April 🎉

**Springtime Doll (or Teddy Bear) Tea.** Decorate in pastels with lots of flowers. Children can "plant" the flowers in small cups as party favors for the doll or teddy bear they bring. Have a contest (with already prepared ribbons or stickers) so that each doll or bear wins a prize for Curliest Hair, Smallest Feet, Pinkest Cheeks, and so on. While the dolls sit somewhere getting acquainted, the children prepare:

**Honey Granola Cookies***
**Lemonade***

This party is fun without any games. Dolls and teddy bears provide the entertainment.

# May 🎉

**Cinco de Mayo Fiesta.** Decorate with the whites, reds, and greens of the flag of Mexico. It would be fun to have a piñata (filled with pennies, small toys, tasty morsels) as a surprise. Talk about this day and compare it to the American Fourth of July. Serve:

**Cheese and Salsa Dip***
**Nachos with a Flourish***
**Cut-up Raw Vegetables**

# June

### Mother's Day or Father's Day or Graduation Supper.
The key here is to save work and have a good time yourself, so fix something super easy:

> **Gingery Barbecue Marinade, poured over chicken the previous night**
> **Baked Potatoes, cooked with chicken**
> **Tossed Green Salad**
> **Peachy-Keen Sundae***

# July

### Fourth of July Party.
Decorate in (what else?) red, white, and blue. If you live in an area that allows fireworks, you can have a twilight party in your own yard. Or you can pack a picnic for an outdoor parade or public fireworks display (see August for picnic ideas). For a good meal that you don't have to grill:

> **Barbecued Anything* (if it's a hot day, use a slow-cooker)**
> **Tomato Tidbits***
> **Raisins on a Log***
> **Mairead's Frozen Treats***
> **Favorite Kid Drinks***

# August

### Dog-Day Picnic or Swim Party.
An outdoor party can be the most fun of all, especially since most of the food is already fixed and the clean-up is easy. Since all three of our children have summer birthdays, we have at least one "sprinkler party" a year. All kids wear bathing suits and play with water balloons or in small wading pools. (Put the largest pool at the bottom of a slide so kids can whoosh into it.) If you're having a beach or pool party, you won't need many games. If you go to a park, try to settle near a shady tree.

### Dog Party or Pet Show:
Just be sure the dogs get along and everybody brings a leash! Snack on:

> **Crazy Carrot Cars***
> **Hard-Boiled Eggs**
> **Carrot Raisin Cookies***
> **Fruit-Cheese Kabobs***
> **Blender Fruit Punch***

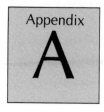

# Appendix A

# HOW TO RUN A FOOD CLUB

- Figure out which items you'd like to carry and make up a sample order form, including weights and prices for all items.
- Ask your friends if they'd like to be included on your mailing list. Also ask for names of others who would be interested in saving money on food.
- Mail out your order form at least a week before customers should turn in their forms and money. Highlight this due date as well as when customers should pick up their orders. For example, mail out order forms on the first of the month, completed requests and money due back to you by the fifteenth, and pick-up a week later.
- Allowing a day or so for late orders, tally how many items you'll order from each distributor and arrange for delivery as close as possible to your pick-up date. You may need to pick up some items yourself if you live in a residential area that forbids truck deliveries.
- On pick-up day, try to have some tasting samples for your customers. We quickly discovered that some chips and salsa, plus the chance to buy just-picked strawberries, made a party atmosphere enjoyed by everybody.
- As with any endeavor, keep your sense of humor. Just as stores face a shortage of goods or late shipments, so can food groups. So if a customer's order of raisins doesn't come in, just smile and ask her if she'd like a credit toward her next order, or the equivalent amount in your extra stock or fresh produce.

During my stint as a food club operator, our young daughters enjoyed seeing how food was sold and loved to sample so many goodies. It was a great form of home schooling, since not many city-raised preschoolers are familiar with grain mills and nut packing plants!

Some final words of experience: new customers come by word of mouth, so don't expect much success from advertising. You may also want to check with your county health department about any local rules for storing and selling of refrigerated items. While a food co-op is usually exempt from such rules, a food club may fall under the requirements for a store.

Over a two-year period, our club grew from 10 to nearly 300 members. And by marking up 20 percent over wholesale prices, we made a small profit in addition to getting all our own food at cost.

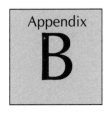

# Appendix B
# RECOMMENDED READINGS AND RESOURCES

*As You Eat So Your Baby Grows*, Nicki Goldbeck; 1978, Cedar Press.

BEANS (Better Educational and Nutritional Standards), promotes local and state legislation about the effects of food on behavior and learning. Write to BEANS, Anastasia Condas, 17766 Hillside Court, Castro Valley, CA 94546.

BIOBOTTOMS, a catalog of natural cotton clothing for newborns through children size 10. Includes cotton diapers, diaper covers, and water-proof cotton bottoms. P.O. Box 1060, 3820 Bodega Avenue, Petaluma, CA 94953.

*Birth Reborn*, Michel Odent. 1986, Pantheon.

*The Book of Whole Grains*, Marlene Anne Bumgarner. 1976, St. Martin's Press.

*The Brown Bag Cookbook*, Sara Sloan. 1984, Williamson.

CENTER FOR SCIENCE IN THE PUBLIC INTEREST. A non-profit group dedicated to consumer health causes, such as the Americans for Safe Food campaign. 1501 Sixteenth Street, N.W., Washington D.C. 20036.

CESAREAN/SUPPORT, EDUCATION AND CONCERN. (C/SEC, Inc.) 22 Forest Road, Framingham, MA 01701.

*Children's Nutrition, A Consumer's Guide*, Lewis A. Coffin. 1984, Capra Press.

*Circumcision: What Every Parent Should Know*, Anne Briggs. 1985, Birth and Parenting.

*A Cooperative Method of Natural Birth Control*, Margaret Nofziger. 1978, Book Publishing Company.

*Diet for a Small Planet*, Frances Moore Lappé. 1982, Ballantine.

*Essential Exercises for the Childbearing Year*, Elizabeth Noble. 1982, Houghton Mifflin.

*The Family Bed*, Tine Thevinin. 1986, Avery.

*The Fast-Food Guide: What's Good, What's Bad, and How To Tell the Difference*, Michael Jacobson and the Center for Science in the Public Interest. 1987.

*Feeding Your Preschool Child*, Karen Olsen. 1986, North Dakota Cooperative Extension Service.

*Feed Your Kids Bright*, Francine and Harold Prince. 1987, Simon and Schuster.

*Feed Your Kids Right*, Lendon Smith, M.D. 1982, Dell.

*Festivals, Family and Food*, Diana Carey and Judy Large. 1982, Hawthorn Press. Available through HearthSong catalog.

*Foods For Healthy Kids*, Lendon Smith, M.D. 1984, Berkeley Books.

*Four Arguments for the Elimination of Television*, Jerry Mander. Morrow.

HEARTHSONG, a catalog for families with goods from all over the globe. High-quality items for children and parents, such as cooking sets, art supplies, lunch baskets, natural foods, and books. P.O. Box B, Sebastopol, CA 95472. (707) 829-1550.

*The Hurried Child: Growing Up Too Fast Too Soon*, David Elkind. 1981, Addison Wesley.

*Jane Brody's Good Food Book*, Jane Brody. 1987, Bantam.

*Jane Brody's Nutrition Book*, Jane Brody. 1987, Bantam.

*If You Love Me, Don't Feed Me Junk!*, Sandy Gooch. 1983, Reston.

*Junk Food, Fast Food, Health Food*, Lila Perl. 1980, Houghton Mifflin.

LA LECHE LEAGUE, a non-profit group dedicated to teaching parents how to give their babies the best start in life by breastfeeding. Look in your phone books for local chapters (who hold monthly meetings and offer free telephone advice) or contact their national headquarters: 9616 Minneapolis Avenue, Franklin Park, IL 60131.

*Let's Have Healthy Children*, Adelle Davis. 1981, New American Library.

*The Magical Child*, Joseph Chilton Pearce. 1980, Bantam.

*Methods of Childbirth*, Constance Bean. 1982, Doubleday.

MUSIC: during labor, can set a soothing and personal tone for the birth. Some suggestions: "Celtic Harp" by Patrick Ball; "Breathe" by Jon Bernoff and Marcus Allen; "As Above So Below" by Kirby Shelstad; "Seascapes" by Michael Jones; "Soft Focus" by Steven Halpern; "Golden Voyage" by Bearns and Dexter; "Miracles" by Rob Whitesides-Woo; "Lullabies From Around the World" by Steve Bergman; and "December" by George Winston.

*Mothering* Magazine, P.O. Box 2208, Albuquerque, NM 87103.

NATIONAL PARENTS-TEACHERS ASSOCIATION, 700 North Rush Street, Chicago, IL 60611-2571.

NATREN, INC., a high-tech producer of cultured milk micronutrients. 10935 Camarillo Street, North Hollywood, CA 91602. Call 1-800-992-9393 in California or 1-800-992-3323 nationally.

*No-Nonsense Nutrition for Kids*, Annette Natow and Jo-Ann Heslin. 1985, Pocket.

*Nursing Your Baby*, Karen Pryor. 1984, Simon & Schuster.

NUTRA PROGRAM, a guide for parents and schools who want good food in their classrooms and cafeterias. P.O. Box 13825, Atlanta, GA 30324.

*Raising Your Child, Not By Force But By Love*, Sidney D. Craig. 1982, Westminster.

*Recipes for a Small Planet*, Ellen Buchman Ewald. 1975, Ballantine.

*A Sigh of Relief, the first-aid handbook for childhood emergencies*, Martin Green. 1977, Bantam.

*Silent Knife*, Nancy Wainer Cohen and Lois J. Estner. 1983, Bergin and Garvey.

*Spiritual Midwifery*, Ina May Gaskin. 1978, The Book Publishing Company.

SUNLIGHT FOODS, a manufacturer of carob and other healthy sweeteners. 2114 Adams Avenue, San Leandro, CA 94577.

SUNRISE AND RAINBOW, a manufacturer of natural supplemental drinks for pregnant and nursing women as well as infants and children to the age of four. In health food stores or order directly: 1-800-826-7957 (CA residents) or 1-800-826-0496.

*The Supermarket Handbook: Access to Whole Foods*, Nikki and David Goldbeck. 1987, New American Library.

*Touching: The Human Significance of Skin*, Ashley Montagu. 1971, Columbia University Press.

UNITED STATES GOVERNMENT PRINTING OFFICE, Consumer Information Catalog, offers many booklets for free or a nominal fee. Some sample booklets: "Consumer's Guide to Food Labels," and "Sweetness Minus Calories Equals Controversy," a discussion of artificial sweeteners. For more information, contact Consumer Information Center-Z, P.O. Box 100, Pueblo, CO 81002.

*the whole birth catalog*, Joy Overbeck. 1986, Pantheon.

*Wise Woman Herbal for the Childbearing Years*, Susun Weed. 1985, Ash Tree.

*Whole Foods for the Whole Family*, La Leche League International Cookbook. 1984, New American Library.

*The Womanly Art of Breastfeeding*, La Leche League International. 1983, New American Library.

# INDEX

## RECIPES ARE INDEXED ON PAGE 232

Sweeteners, 84–86
Sweets, 66, 82–87, 103–4, 149
Swim party, 225

Teddy bear tea, 224
Teething, 60, 67, 70, 78
Thevinin, Tine, 35
Thompson, Marian, 42, 88
Toddler, 75–93
Tooth decay, 87
Toxemia, 11

United States Food and Drug Administration, 138

Valentine's Day party, 224
Vegetables, 10, 23, 100–102, 109, 123, 128
Vegetarian diets, 22, 111
Virtue, Joyce, 70–72

Vitamins
  A, 55
  allergies and, 72
  B, 14, 16, 43, 78, 85–87, 124
  breastmilk and, 5
  C, 9, 23, 78, 124
  E, 14, 43
  empty calories and, 108
  first foods and, 65
  K, 43
  postnatal diet and, 43
  prenatal, 9
  supplements, 15–18, 55–56, 78, 124
Vomiting, 38

Weaning, 87–92
Weight gain, 10–13, 79, 105–6
Weintraub, Denis, 56
Weiss, Ted, 138
Wenner, Paul, 136
White flour, 18, 84

Young, Frank E., 138

# RECIPE INDEX

Alphabet recipes, 215–20
Appetizers, 173–76
Apples
  applesauce from a blender, 216
  applesauce whip, 202
  baked apples, 164
  breakfast apple cobbler, 153
  carob-coated apples, 202
  surprise apple pancakes, 157
Artichokes
  chunky artichoke casserole, 174–75
  cold artichoke hearts, 164

Baby foods. See First foods
Barbecue sauce, 178
Beans
  bean filling, 179

beaned-out casserole, 180
leftover beans sandwiches, 163
make your own burger, 183
nachos, 184–85
pumpkin pot stew, 186–87
slow-cooker beans, 187
sprouts, 167
Beverages, 195–99
Bones for teething, 146
Breads, 191–94
Breakfasts, 156–58, 199
Burritos, 179, 183

Cake
  almond coffee cake, 152
  Irish gingerbread, 209
Cantaloupe, 147